改訂新版

これだけは知っておきたい
看護英語の基本用語と表現

NURSING
TERMS AND EXPRESSIONS
EVERYBODY USES

編著者
園城寺康子　川越栄子

英文校閲
Christine D. Kuramoto

MEDICAL VIEW

Nursing Terms and Expressions Everybody Uses, 2nd edition
(ISBN978-4-7583-0446-7 C3047)

Editors:	Yasuko Onjohji
	Eiko Kawagoe
English Advisor:	Christine D. Kuramoto

2007. 3.30 1st ed.
2016. 1.10 2nd ed.

©MEDICAL VIEW, 2007 & 2016
Printed and Bound in Japan

Medical View Co., Ltd.

2-30 Ichigaya-honmuracho, Shinjuku-ku, Tokyo 162-0845, Japan
E-mail ed@medicalview.co.jp

改訂新版刊行にあたって

 2007年に『これだけは知っておきたい 看護英語の基本用語と表現』が刊行されてから9年が経過しました。その間,医療・看護を取り巻く環境は大きく変化しています。

 訪日外国人数は,2007年には約800万人でしたが,2015年には2,000万人に届こうとしています。それに伴い,訪日中に医療機関を訪れる外国人数が激増しています。2020年のオリンピックにおいても多くの外国人が訪日することが予想されます。訪日外国人と在留外国人(約200万人)の患者さんに対して,医療従事者は世界共通語である英語で対応できることが求められています。また,超高齢化社会に突入する日本においては,質の高い医療・看護や高度な専門知識が求められるため,英語論文から世界の情報を得ることも必要になっています。

 そのような医療・看護を取り巻く環境に対応できるように,改訂新版では,看護英語を3つのパートに分けました。PART 1「主な看護分野の基本用語と表現」では主な看護専門7分野の基本用語 約980語と基本表現 約170例,PART 2「病棟で使われる基本用語と表現」では基本用語 約550語と基本表現 約280例,PART 3「解剖・徴候・疾患の基本用語と表現」では基本用語 約1,050語と基本表現 約270例を掲載しました。これらをマスターすれば,専門職として質の高いケアを英語で行うのに困らないように配慮いたしました。

 また,それぞれのPartの各セクションでは,「基本用語」と「基本表現」がセットになっていて,用語を学習しながら実際に使える表現を身に付けられるように工夫しています。

 このように,新たな医療環境のニーズに合わせて本書が改訂新版として刊行される運びになりました。国内・国外の多くの患者さんをサポートするために役立てていただけることを編著者一同願ってやみません。

2015年10月　　編著者

初版刊行にあたって

　1998年に「これだけは知っておきたい医学英語の基本用語と表現」(藤枝宏壽, 玉巻欣子, Randolph Mann編著) が刊行され大変好評を得ています。今回その姉妹編として本書を刊行させていただく事になりました。医療界は大きく変化し, 看護職員が臨床の場で外国人に対応し, また看護学の研究者として英語で論文を発表する事が求められる時代になっています。そのために最低限必要な英語の用語と表現を身に付けておくことが不可欠になっています。それらのニーズに合わせて本書が刊行される運びになりました。

　看護英語は医学英語と重なる部分もありますが, 患者さんの生活をサポートする語彙・表現を中心に看護特有のものがあります。そのような日々のケアに必要な語彙をPart I「日常医療英語の語彙」に主に名詞を約2100語, Part III「ケアにおける日常表現」に必要な表現を約450個まとめ, これらをマスターすれば英語でケアするには困らないように配慮いたしました。また, これらの用語は看護英語論文講読・執筆に必要な用語であることはいうまでもありません。

　特に本書で「日常生活のストレスと悩み」「患者の日常生活」を入れたのは, ストレスの多い現代社会におけるケアの場で重要な用語であるからです。また従来の用語集には少なかった「公衆衛生」「終末期ケアと死」を充実させ現代医療のニーズに対応できるようにしました。

　さらに本書独自の特徴としてPart II「国際化に対応するための語彙」に看護職員として国際的に活躍するために必要な用語を集めました。これらの用語リストはまだ他書には例を見ないものです。「看護行為」の動詞はICNP (International Classification for Nursing Practice：看護実践国際分類) を参考に国際的基準に照らして看護に必要な動詞をまとめました。動詞は看護英語を理解するうえでPart Iの名詞に次いで重要なものです。「看護関連用語」「看護専門分野」「国際看護」は, 看護学の研究者として世界の研究者と共に研究を進めるうえで, また国

際保健活動に参加する際に必要となる用語です。さらに、「アメリカ国家試験頻出用語」を加えました。アメリカでの正看護師（Registered Nurse）免許の取得方法は州によって異なりますが、一般にNCLEX-RN（National Council of Licensure Examination for Registered Nurses）と呼ばれる看護師試験に合格する必要があります。当試験に出る頻出用語をまとめました。

　看護の世界にも国際化の波が押し寄せていますが、この新しい時代に対応できるように本書は産声を上げました。看護職者として世界へ大きく飛び立つ人たちの第一歩に役立つ事を編著者一同願ってやみません。

2007年3月　　編著者

PART 1　主な看護分野の基本用語と表現

1-01　Adult Nursing　成人看護　　2

Words and Terms　基本用語　2
1. General Terms：一般用語　2
2. Diseases, Treatments：疾患と治療　5
3. Supplies and Equipment：用品と器具　6
4. Stressful Life Events：ストレスになる出来事　6
5. Related Terms：その他　7

Expressions　表現　8

1-02　Pediatric Nursing　小児看護　　10

Words and Terms　基本用語　10
1. General Terms：一般用語　10
2. Diseases, Treatments：疾患と治療　11
3. Newborn and Infant Care：新生児と幼児のケア　13

Expressions　表現　15

1-03　Psychiatric Nursing　精神看護　　16

Words and Terms　基本用語　16
1. General Terms：一般用語　16
2. Diseases, Treatments：疾患と治療　17
3. Stressful Life Events：ストレスになる出来事　18

Expressions　表現　20

1-04　Maternal Nursing　母性看護　　21

Words and Terms　基本用語　21
1. Pregnancy：妊娠　21
2. Childbirth：出産　22
3. Childcare：育児　24
4. Diseases, Treatments：疾患と治療　25
5. Related Terms：その他　26

Expressions　表現　28

- ① Pregnancy：妊娠 ………………………………28
- ② Childbirth：出産 ………………………………29
- ③ Childcare：育児 ………………………………30
- ④ Women's Health：ウィメンズヘルス …………31

1-05 Community Health Nursing 地域看護　32

Words and Terms 基本用語 ………………………32
- ① Community Health Nursing：地域看護 ………32
- ② School Health：学校保健 ……………………33
- ③ Stressful Life Events：ストレスになる出来事 …34
- ④ Related Terms：その他 ………………………35

Expressions 表現 ………………………………36

1-06 Geriatric Nursing 老年看護　37

Words and Terms 基本用語 ………………………37
- ① General Terms：一般用語 ……………………37
- ② Diseases, Treatments：疾患と治療 …………38
- ③ Nursing Concerns：患者さんへの配慮 ………39
- ④ Terminal Care and Death：終末期ケアと死 …39

Expressions 表現 ………………………………43

1-07 Home Care Nursing 在宅看護　45

Words and Terms 基本用語 ………………………45

Expressions 表現 ………………………………47

1-08 Fundamental Nursing 基礎看護　50

Words and Terms 基本用語 ………………………50
- ① Insurance and Health Care Financing：
  健康保険関連用語 ………………………………50
- ② Public Health：公衆衛生 ………………………50
- ③ Nursing Care Planning 看護計画関連用語 …55
- ④ Nursing Specialties 看護専門分野 …………56

Expressions 表現 ………………………………59

PART 2　病棟で使われる基本用語と表現

2-01　Facility　病院施設　　62

Words and Terms　基本用語　62
1. Ward, Unit：病棟　62
2. Outpatient Department：外来　63
3. Patient's Room：病室　64
4. Other Areas：その他のエリア　64
5. Nursing Supplies：看護用品　65
6. Equipment for Care：看護機器　67

Expressions　表現　70
1. 入院準備：Preparation for Hospitalization　70
2. 入院生活：Life in Hospital　71
3. 退院：Discharge　73
4. Operation：手術　74
5. Daily Routine：日常生活　78

2-02　Hospital Personnel　医療従事者　　81

Words and Terms　基本用語　81
1. Administrators：管理職　81
2. Nursing Department：看護部　81
3. Physician and Staff：医師, スタッフ　82
4. Areas of Specialty and Specialists：専門と専門医　83

Expressions　表現　85
1. Reception：受付　85
2. Registration and Personal Profile：登録, 個人情報　86
3. Hospital Guide：院内案内　87

2-03 Medications 薬剤 … 92

Words and Terms 基本用語 … 92
- ❶ General Terms：一般用語 … 92
- ❷ Route of Administration：形態，用法 … 94
- ❸ Types of Medications：薬の種類 … 95

Expressions 表現 … 97

2-04 Daily Activities of Patients 患者さんの日常生活 … 99

Words and Terms 基本用語 … 99
- ❶ Daily Actions：日々の行為 … 99
- ❷ Eating：食事 … 99
- ❸ Grooming and Cleanliness：身づくろい … 101
- ❹ Excretion：排泄 … 102
- ❺ Sleep：睡眠 … 103
- ❻ Personal Belongings：身周り品 … 103
- ❼ Others：その他 … 104

Expressions 表現 … 105
- ❶ Eating：食事 … 105
- ❷ Excretion：排泄 … 106
- ❸ Bathing 入浴 … 107
- ❹ Sleep：睡眠 … 108

PART 3　解剖・徴候・疾患の基本用語と表現

3-01　External Body Parts 身体の外部 … 112
Words and Terms 基本用語 … 112
Expressions 表現 … 115

3-02　Internal Body Parts 身体の内部 … 116
Words and Terms 基本用語 … 116
1. Skeletal System：骨格系 … 116
2. Muscular and Joint System：筋, 関節系 … 117
3. Brain and Nervous System：脳, 神経系 … 117
4. Respiratory System：呼吸器系 … 118
5. Circulatory System：循環器系 … 118
6. Digestive System：消化器系 … 119
7. Urinary and Reproductive Systems：
   腎・泌尿器, 生殖器系 … 119
8. Ear, Nose, Throat and Eye：耳, 鼻, 咽喉, 眼 … 120
9. Skin：皮膚 … 121
10. Dentistry：歯科 … 121
11. Endocrine System：内分泌系 … 122
12. Blood and Immune System：血液, 免疫系 … 122

Expressions 表現 … 123
1. Skeletal System：骨格系 … 123
2. Muscular and Joint System：筋, 関節系 … 123
3. Brain and Nervous System：脳, 神経系 … 124
4. Respiratory System：呼吸器系 … 124
5. Circulatory System：循環器系 … 125
6. Digestive System：消化器系 … 126
7. Urinary and Reproductive Systems：
   腎・泌尿器, 生殖器系 … 127
8. Ear, Nose, Throat and Eye：耳, 鼻, 咽喉, 眼 … 128
9. Skin：皮膚 … 130
10. Dentistry：歯科 … 131

- ⑪ Endocrine System：内分泌系 ··················132
- ⑫ Blood and Immune System：血液，免疫系 ···133

3-03 Symptoms 症候と徴候　　134

Words and Terms 基本用語 ························134
- ① General Symptoms：一般的な症候 ···········134
- ② Bone, Muscle, Joint：骨，筋，関節 ············136
- ③ Brain and Nervous System：脳，神経系 ·····136
- ④ Respiratory System：呼吸器系 ················137
- ⑤ Circulatory System：循環器系 ·················137
- ⑥ Digestive System：消化器系 ···················138
- ⑦ Kidney and Urinary System：腎・泌尿器系 ···139
- ⑧ Ear, Nose, Throat and Eye：耳，鼻，咽喉，眼 ···139
- ⑨ Skin：皮膚 ···140
- ⑩ Dentistry：歯科 ·····································141
- ⑪ Frequency：症状の頻度 ··························142
- ⑫ Intensity：症状の強さ ·····························142
- ⑬ Types of Pain：痛みの種類 ······················143

Expressions 表現 ·······································144
- ① 健康上の習慣：Health Habits ···················144
- ② 排泄，生理：Excretion, Menstrual Period ···146

3-04 Diseases, Conditions and Wounds 疾患と創傷　　147

Words and Terms 基本用語 ························147
- ① Bone, Muscle, Joint：骨，筋，関節 ············147
- ② Brain and Nervous System：脳，神経系 ·····147
- ③ Respiratory System：呼吸器系 ················148
- ④ Circulatory System：循環器系 ·················148
- ⑤ Digestive System：消化器系 ···················149
- ⑥ Kidney and Urinary System：腎・泌尿器系 ···149
- ⑦ Ear, Nose, Throat and Eye：耳，鼻，咽喉，眼 ···150
- ⑧ Skin：皮膚 ···151

- ❾ Dentistry：歯科 ･･････････････････････152
- ❿ Endocrine System：内分泌系 ････････････152
- ⓫ Blood and Immune System：血液，免疫系 ･･････152
- ⓬ Infectious Diseases：感染症 ･･････････････152
- **Expressions** 表現 ･････････････････････154

3-05 Diagnostic Tests 検査　155

Words and Terms 基本用語 ･･･････････････155
- ❶ Common Tests：一般的な検査 ･･････････155
- ❷ Bone, Muscle, Joint：骨，筋，関節 ･･･････156
- ❸ Brain and Nervous System：脳，神経系 ･･･156
- ❹ Respiratory System：呼吸器系 ･････････156
- ❺ Circulatory System：循環器系 ･･････････157
- ❻ Digestive System：消化器系 ･･･････････157
- ❼ Kidney and Urinary System：腎・泌尿器系 ･･158
- ❽ Ear, Nose, Throat and Eye：耳，鼻，咽喉，眼 ･･158
- ❾ Endocrine System：内分泌系 ････････････158
- ❿ Blood：血液 ･･････････････････････････159
- ⓫ Equipment and Supplies：検査機器 ･････162

Expressions 表現 ･････････････････････163
- ❶ Blood Test：血液検査 ･････････････････163
- ❷ Collecting Urine and Stool Specimens：
  尿検査，便検査 ･･････････････････････163
- ❸ EKG, etc.：心電図など ････････････････164

3-06 Physical Examination 診察　166

Words and Terms 基本用語 ･･･････････････166
- ❶ General Terms：一般用語 ･･･････････････166
- ❷ Vital Signs：バイタルサイン ････････････167
- ❸ Physical Check-up：健康診断 ･･･････････168

Expressions 表現 ･････････････････････170
- ❶ Blood Pressure：血圧 ･････････････････170
- ❷ Body Temperature：体温 ･･････････････170

3-07 Treatment and Therapy 治療と療法　171

Words and Terms 基本用語 ・・・・・・・・・・・・・・・・・・・・・・・・171
- ❶ Treatment and Operations：治療と手術 ・・・・・・・・・171
- ❷ Therapies：療法 ・・・・・・・・・・・・・・・・・・・・・・・・・・・・・・172
- ❸ Posture, Position：体位 ・・・・・・・・・・・・・・・・・・・・・・・175

Expressions 表現 ・・・・・・・・・・・・・・・・・・・・・・・・・・・・・・・176
- ❶ 注射，点滴：Injection, IV ・・・・・・・・・・・・・・・・・・・・・176
- ❷ 包帯など：Bandage, etc. ・・・・・・・・・・・・・・・・・・・・・・177
- ❸ 体位など：Body Position, etc. ・・・・・・・・・・・・・・・・・178

Index
日本語索引 ・・・・179
英語索引 ・・・・・・204
略語索引 ・・・・・・231

コラム

| 赤ちゃん言葉 ・・・・14 | ことわざ1 ・・・・・・・27 | 心のケア ・・・・・・・・42 |
| 看護雑誌の略称 ・・58 | °F/°C換算 ・・・・・・69 | ことわざ2 ・・・・・・104 |

本書の使い方

(1) 重要な語彙は太字にしています。まずそれらの重要語から覚えていってください。
(2) 学生なら教科書の英語でわからない語句があったとき，すでに看護職についている人ならカルテに書かれている英語でわからなかった場合，索引を使って本書を辞書がわりに使ってください。

謝　辞

　姉妹編としての出版をご快諾いただいた藤枝宏壽先生，玉巻欣子先生，Randolph Mann 先生に感謝申し上げるとともに，適切な御助言をいただいた神戸市看護大学・聖路加国際大学の諸先生に心から感謝の意を表します。

統一表記

太字	基本的な単語
( )	「または」の意；直前の語と入れ替えてよい。 例 瞼(まぶた)，delivery table (stand)
〔 〕	省略可能 例 高血圧〔症〕，〔a pair of〕slippers
[ ]	略語 例 tuberculin reaction [TR]
/	対応する語 例 lower lid / upper lip → 下まぶた／上まぶた
;	語の区切 例 navel; belly button; umbilicus
斜体	ラテン語 例 *in vitro*

PART 1
主な看護分野の基本用語と表現

Adult Nursing

成人看護

Words and Terms 基本用語

① General Terms：一般用語

1. ☐ outpatient nursing — 外来看護
2. ☐ **cancer nursing** — **がん看護**
3. ☐ **family nursing** — **家族看護**
4. ☐ disaster nursing — 災害看護
5. ☐ certified social worker — 社会福祉士
6. ☐ psychiatric social worker — 精神保健福祉士
7. ☐ paramedic — 救急医療隊員
8. ☐ clinical psychologist — 臨床心理士
9. ☐ clinical engineer[CE] — 臨床工学技士
10. ☐ medical policy — 医療政策
11. ☐ health statistics — 保健統計学
12. ☐ industrial hygiene — 産業保健
13. ☐ primary care — プライマリーケア
14. ☐ acute medical care — 急性期医療
15. ☐ infection management — 感染管理
16. ☐ hospital infection — 院内感染
17. ☐ infection control — 感染予防
18. ☐ preventive medicine — 予防医学
19. ☐ resuscitation — 救急蘇生
20. ☐ relief technique — 救護技術
21. ☐ malpractice — 医療過誤, 医療事故
22. ☐ informed consent — インフォームド・コンセント

成人看護

1	☐ counseling	カウンセリング
2	☐ conference	カンファレンス
3	☐ second opinion	セカンドオピニオン
4	☐ right of self-determination; autonomy	自己決定権
6	☐ **pain management**	**疼痛管理**
7	☐ **tube feeding**	**経管栄養法**
8	☐ vital signs[VS]	バイタルサイン
9	☐ triage	トリアージ
10	☐ cyanosis	チアノーゼ
11	☐ allergic reaction	アレルギー反応
12	☐ advanced medical care	先進医療
13	☐ organ transplantation	臓器移植
14	☐ brain death	脳死
15	☐ metabolic syndrome	メタボリックシンドローム
16	☐ clinical nutrition	病態栄養
17	☐ certified health food	保健機能食品
18	☐ frigidity	不感症
19	☐ sexual debility	性欲減退
20	☐ sexual impotence; erectile dysfunction[ED]	ペニス勃起不能, 性的不能
22	☐ libido	性欲
23	☐ mental health	メンタルヘルス
24	☐ health assessment	ヘルスアセスメント
25	☐ physical assessment	フィジカルアセスメント
26	☐ enema	浣腸
27	☐ suppository	坐薬
28	☐ depilation	脱毛
29	☐ blood transfusion	輸血
30	☐ feeding tube diet	経管栄養剤

PART1　主な看護分野の基本用語と表現

1	☐ catheterization	カテーテル法
2	☐ catheter obstruction	カテーテル閉塞
3	☐ gastric fistula,	胃瘻
4	gastrostoma	
5	☐ nasogastric tube feeding	経鼻胃管栄養法
6	☐ stoma	ストーマ
7	☐ self-catheterization	自己導尿
8	☐ insulin	インスリン
9	☐ body mass index[BMI]	体格指数
10	☐ peritoneal dialysis[PD]	腹膜透析法
11	☐ intravenous hyperalimentation[IVH]	中心静脈栄養法
12		
13	☐ total parenteral nutrition [TPN]	完全静脈栄養
14		
15	☐ drug therapy monitoring	服薬管理
16	☐ noninvasive positive pressure ventilation [NPPV]	非侵襲的陽圧換気
17		
18		
19	☐ lubricating topical anesthetic	潤滑剤表面麻酔剤
20		
21	☐ living will	リビング・ウィル
22	☐ total pain	全人的苦痛(トータルペイン)
23	☐ **grief care**	悲嘆回復(グリーフケア)
24	☐ protection of privacy	プライバシーの保護
25	☐ relaxation	リラクゼーション
26	☐ visiting	面会
27	☐ discharge guidance	退院指導
28	☐ **discharge support**	退院支援

② Diseases, Treatments：疾患と治療

1. ☐ disorder — 障害
2. ☐ intractable disease — 難病
3. ☐ dysphagia — 嚥下障害
4. ☐ abdominal bloating — 腹部膨満
5. ☐ hypoglycemia — 低血糖
6. ☐ hyperglycemia — 高血糖
7. ☐ food poisoning — 食中毒
8. ☐ delirium — せん妄
9. ☐ blood clot — 血の塊
10. ☐ complication — 合併症
11. ☐ sequela — 続発症
12. ☐ contagious disease — 伝染病
13. ☐ **acute disease** — **急性疾患**
14. ☐ **chronic disease** — **慢性疾患**
15. ☐ family (hereditary; inherited) disease — 遺伝病
17. ☐ malnutrition — 栄養失調〔症〕
18. ☐ amyotrophic lateral sclerosis［ALS］— 筋萎縮性側索硬化症
20. ☐ Parkinson's disease — パーキンソン病
21. ☐ epilepsy — てんかん
22. ☐ dehydration — 脱水症
23. ☐ diarrhea — 下痢
24. ☐ constipation — 便秘
25. ☐ catheter infection — カテーテル感染症
26. ☐ life-prolonging treatment — 延命治療
27. ☐ chemotherapy — 化学療法
28. ☐ radiation therapy — 放射線療法

1	☐ multimodal treatment	集学的治療
2	☐ dietetic treatment	食事療法
3	☐ tracheostomy	気管切開
4	☐ oral care	口腔ケア

③ Supplies and Equipment：用品と器具

7	☐ **wheelchair**	車椅子
8	☐ artificial limb	義肢
9	☐ **walker**	**歩行器**
10	☐ positioning aids	体位変換器
11	☐ braille writer	点字器
12	☐ artificial larynx	人工喉頭
13	☐ cast immobilization	ギプス固定
14	☐ brace wearing	装具装着
15	☐ feeding tube	栄養チューブ
16	☐ irrigator	イリゲーター
17	☐ syringe	注射器
18	☐ injection needle	注射針
19	☐ pulse oximeter	パルスオキシメーター
20	☐ automated external defibrillator [AED]	自動体外式除細動器

④ Stressful Life Events：ストレスになる出来事

24	☐ lost love	失恋
25	☐ breakup with a lover	恋人との別れ
26	☐ trouble with superiors	上司とのトラブル
27	☐ restructuring	リストラ
28	☐ unemployment	失業
29	☐ debt	借金
30	☐ mortgage	住宅ローン

1	☐ bankruptcy	破産
2	☐ death of one's child	子どもの死
3	☐ husband's (wife's) unfaithfulness; cheating	夫(妻)の浮気
5	☐ traffic accident	交通事故
6	☐ breakup of one's marriage	結婚の破たん
8	☐ separation	別居
9	☐ divorce	離婚
10	☐ illness of a family member	家族の病気
12	☐ retirement	退職
13	☐ being employed/ unemployed	就職／無職
15	☐ marriage	結婚
16	☐ remarriage	再婚
17	☐ pregnancy	妊娠
18	☐ childbirth	出産
19	☐ home-buying	住宅購入
20	☐ starting a business	事業の開始
21	☐ promotion	昇進
22	☐ moving	引越し
23	☐ empty nest	子どもの独立

⑤ Related Terms：その他

26	☐ multiple	多発性の
27	☐ **benign**	**良性の**
28	☐ **malignant**	**悪性の**
29	☐ congenital	先天性の
30	☐ acquired	後天性の

Expressions 表現

①心配しないでください。大丈夫ですよ。
  Don't worry. It's all right now (It will be all right / You'll be all right).

②ご気分はいかがですか。
  How are you feeling?

③どうぞ落ち着いてください。もう大丈夫ですよ。
  Please relax. Please stay calm. You'll be OK.

④あわてないでください。
  Please don't panic.

⑤いつでもお気軽になんでも聞いてください。
  Please feel free to ask any questions.

⑥もう少し食べましょう。元気が出ますよ。
  Try to eat a little more. It will give you energy.

⑦今日は調子がよさそうですね。
  You look fine today.

⑧早くお元気になってください。
  I hope you will get well soon.

⑨あきらめないでください。
  Don't give up.

⑩気を楽にしてください。
  Take it easy.

⑪すぐによくなりますよ。
  You'll feel better soon.

⑫順調ですよ。
  You're doing fine.

⑬2〜3分で済みますから。
  It'll be over in a few minutes.

⑭すぐによくなるといいですね。
I hope you'll feel better soon.

⑮よくわかります。
I see.
I understand.

⑯どうかあまり心配しないようにしてください。
Please try not to worry so much.

⑰どうぞお大事にしてください。
Please take good care of yourself.

⑱それはお気の毒に。
That's too bad.

⑲何か私にできることがありますか。
What can I do for you?

⑳大変だったのですね。
That must have been really hard (tough).

㉑とてもおつらいでしょうね。
This must be (have been) very hard for you.

㉒また後でお話しましょう。
I'll talk with you later.

㉓どうなさいましたか。何かご心配ですか。
What is worrying you?
What are you concerned about?

㉔もう少し詳しく話してくださいますか。
Can you tell me more about it?

㉕しばらくおそばについています。
I'll be (sit) with you for a while.

Pediatric Nursing

小児看護

Words and Terms　基本用語

① General Terms：一般用語

#		
1	☐ **developmental nursing**	発達看護
2	☐ growth support	生育支援
3	☐ live birth	生児出生
4	☐ **neonate**	新生児
5	☐ **fetus**	胎児
6	☐ fetal monitoring	胎児モニタリング
7	☐ fetal heart rate	胎児心拍
8	☐ development of fetus	胎児の発達
9	☐ weight gain	体重増加
10	☐ low birth weight [LBW]	低出生体重
11-12	☐ extremely low birth weight infant	超低出生体重児
13	☐ fetal distress	胎児仮死
14	☐ high risk infant	ハイリスク児
15-16	☐ neonatal behavioral assessment scale [NBAS]	新生児行動評価
17	☐ Apgar score	アプガースコア
18	☐ nurture	療育
19-20	☐ stroke; fit; ictus; insult; attack; seizure; paroxysm	発作
21-22	☐ neonatal intensive care unit [NICU]	新生児集中治療室

1	☐ school for children with disabilities	養護学校
3	☐ hospital school	院内学級
4	☐ independence support	自立支援
5	☐ school nurse	養護教諭
6	☐ intermittent self-catheterization	間欠自己導尿
8	☐ toilet training	トイレトレーニング
9	☐ bedwetting	寝小便
10	☐ defecation reflex	排便反射
11	☐ primitive reflex	原始反射
12	☐ itching sensation	搔痒感
13	☐ moisturizer	保湿剤
14	☐ steroid	ステロイド
15	☐ tuberculin reaction [TR]	ツベルクリン反応

② Diseases, Treatments：疾患と治療

18	☐ **mumps**	**おたふく風邪**
19	☐ **measles**	**はしか**
20	☐ rubella	風疹
21	☐ polio	ポリオ, 小児麻痺
22	☐ **chickenpox, varicella**	**水痘**
23	☐ pertussis	百日咳
24	☐ colic	〔子供の〕疝痛, 激しい腹痛
25	☐ atopic dermatitis	アトピー性皮膚炎
26	☐ food allergy	食物アレルギー
27	☐ febrile convulsion	熱性けいれん
28	☐ 〔infant〕respiratory distress syndrome [RDS]	呼吸窮迫症候群
30	☐ intellectually disabled	精神遅滞

1	☐ **learning disabilities [LD]**	学習障害
2	☐ Down's syndrome	ダウン症候群
3	☐ Turner's syndrome	ターナー症候群
4	☐ **attention deficit hyperactivity disorder [ADHD]**	注意欠陥過活動性障害
7	☐ failure to thrive	成長障害
8	☐ cleft lip	口唇裂
9	☐ cleft palate	口蓋裂
10	☐ neonatal hypoglycemia	新生児低血糖
11	☐ hypogonadism	性腺機能低下症
12	☐ congenital esophageal atresia	先天性食道閉鎖症
14	☐ congenital hip dislocation	先天性股関節脱臼
15	☐ sudden infant death syndrome [SIDS]	乳幼児突然死亡症候群
17	☐ childhood cancer	小児がん
18	☐ leukemia	白血病
19	☐ acute lymphocytic leukemia [ALL]	急性リンパ性白血病
21	☐ brain tumor	脳腫瘍
22	☐ hydrocephalus	水頭症
23	☐ childhood bronchial asthma	小児気管支喘息
25	☐ airway obstruction	気道閉塞
26	☐ airway management	気道確保
27	☐ allergen elimination	アレルゲン除去
28	☐ growth hormone treatment	成長ホルモン治療

	cardiopulmonary resuscitation [CPR]	心肺蘇生
	newborn resuscitation	新生児蘇生

③ Newborn and Infant Care：新生児と幼児のケア

	infant	幼児
	premature baby	未熟児
	baby boy / baby girl	男の赤ちゃん／女の赤ちゃん
	bonding	きずな
	baby talk	赤ちゃん言葉
	babbling	〔赤ちゃんの〕片言
	fuss	ぐずる
	crawl	はいはい歩きする
	drool	よだれをたらす
	hold up one's head	首がすわる
	grasp	ギュッと握る
	dehydration	脱水
	shivering	ふるえ
	diaper rash	オムツかぶれ
	heat rash	あせも
	teething	乳歯が生えること
	finger sucking	指しゃぶり
	cuddle	抱きしめる
	medical checkup	**健診**
	immunization; shot; vaccination	**予防注射**
	well-baby clinic [WBC]	育児相談
	incubator	保育器, 保温器
	Apgar score	アプガースコア
	fontanelle; soft spot	泉門 (前頭部の柔らかい部分)

1-02 Pediatric Nursing

1. ☐ baby bottle — 哺乳瓶
2. ☐ baby food — 離乳食
3. ☐ bottle feeding — 人工栄養
4. ☐ formula — 乳児用ミルク
5. ☐ nipple of baby bottle — 哺乳瓶の乳首
6. ☐ breast milk — 母乳
7. ☐ breast feeding — 母乳栄養
8. ☐ breast binder — 〔母乳で張ったときの〕胸当て
9. ☐ security blanket — お守り毛布(ねんねタオル)
10. ☐ toy — おもちゃ

---

column 赤ちゃん言葉

日本語には「わんわん」「あんよ」のような赤ちゃん言葉がありますが，英語も同じように幼児に使う言葉があります。少し例をあげておきます。小さい子供をケアするときに使ってください。

ぽんぽん（腹）tummy おへそ tummy-button
あんよ（足）footsie おてて pud
おしっこ pee-pee おちんちん wee-wee
わんわん（犬）bowwow にゃんにゃん（猫）kitty
お人形さん dolly おしゃぶり passy; pacifier
毛布 blankie パジャマ jammie
こちょこちょ coochy-coochy-coo

Expressions 表現

①お嬢ちゃんはどうしましたか。
What is her problem?

②ミルクを飲みますか。
Does he/she drink milk?

③お子さんはどのくらいの頻度でおしっこをしますか。
How often does he/she pass water?

④便は何色ですか。
What color is his/her stool?

⑤お子さんはよくぐずりますか。
Does he/she often cry?

⑥おりこうさんだね。
Good girl (boy) !

⑦ぽんぽんが痛いかな。
Does your tummy hurt?

⑧大丈夫だよ。
It will be all right.

⑨心配しないで。
Don't worry.

⑩すぐ終わるよ。
It will be over soon.

⑪そばにいるからね。
I'll stay with you.

⑫痛くないよ。
It's not going to hurt.

Psychiatric Nursing

精神看護

Words and Terms　基本用語

① General Terms：一般用語

1	☐ **mental care**	**心のケア**
2	☐ listening	傾聴
3	☐ **mental health**	**心の健康**
4	☐ social withdrawal	引きこもり
5	☐ forgetfulness	もの忘れ
6	☐ adult children	アダルト・チルドレン
7	☐ mentally challenged person	精神障害者
9	☐ dependence	依存症
10	☐ codependency	共依存
11	☐ suicidal ideation	希死念慮
12	☐ suicidal wishes	自殺願望
13	☐ suicide attempt	自殺企図
14	☐ suicide	自殺
15	☐ self-injury	自傷
16	☐ psychogenic	心因性の
17	☐ prodromal period	前駆期
18	☐ independence support	自立支援
19	☐ Mental Health Act	精神保健福祉法
20	☐ Services and Support for People with Disabilities Act	障害者自立支援法

精神看護

1	☐ Medical Treatment and Supervision Act	医療観察法
3	☐ adult guardianship	成年後見制度
4	☐ disability support services center	障害者地域生活支援センター
6	☐ daily living training center	生活訓練施設
7	☐ vocational aid center	授産施設
8	☐ drug abuse	薬物乱用
9	☐ **sleeping pill**	**睡眠薬**
10	☐ **tranquilizer**	**精神安定剤**
11	☐ **sedative**	**鎮静剤**
12	☐ antidepressant	抗うつ剤
13	☐ neurotropic drug	向神経薬
14	☐ psychotropic drug	向精神薬

② Diseases, Treatments：疾患と治療

17	☐ **mental disease**	**精神疾患**
18	☐ depression	うつ病, 憂うつ, 抑うつ
19	☐ bipolar disorder; manic depression	躁うつ病
21	☐ mania	躁病
22	☐ mood disorder	気分障害
23	☐ developmental disorder	発達障害
24	☐ anxiety disorder	不安障害
25	☐ alcoholism	アルコール依存症
26	☐ eating disorder	摂食障害
27	☐ anorexia 〔nervosa〕	神経性食欲不振症(拒食症)
28	☐ bulimia 〔nervosa〕	過食症
29	☐ schizophrenia	統合失調症
30	☐ nervous breakdown	神経衰弱

1	☐ dementia	認知症
2	☐ neurosis	ノイローゼ, 神経症
3	☐ anxiety neurosis	不安神経症
4	☐ autism	自閉症
5	☐ post traumatic stress disorder[PTSD]	心的外傷後ストレス障害
7	☐ psychosomatic disorder	心身症
8	☐ **insomnia**	**不眠症**
9	☐ hysteria	ヒステリー症
10	☐ cognitive behavioral therapy	認知行動療法
12	☐ family therapy	家族療法
13	☐ interpersonal psychotherapy[IPT]	対人関係療法
15	☐ psychiatric pharmacotherapy	精神科薬物療法
17	☐ psychological first aid [PFA]	サイコロジカルファーストエイド

③ **Stressful Life Events**：ストレスになる出来事

21	☐ **stress**	ストレス
22	☐ anxiety	不安
23	☐ fear	恐怖
24	☐ threat	脅威
25	☐ a deep emotional scar; feeling troubled	心の闇
27	☐ fretfulness	焦り
28	☐ loneliness	孤独
29	☐ alienation	疎外感

1	intense self-consciousness	自意識過剰
3	self-esteem	自尊心
4	conflict	葛藤
5	discomfort	不快
6	anger	怒り
7	irritation	いらだち
8	hatred	憎しみ
9	grudge	怨恨
10	heaviness	重苦しさ
11	grief	悲しみ
12	excitement	興奮
13	panic	パニック
14	manic state	躁状態
15	fear of other people	対人恐怖
16	social isolation	社会的孤立
17	neglect	ネグレクト
18	**abuse**	**虐待**
19	**domestic violence [DV]**	**家庭内暴力**
20	alcohol dependence	アルコール依存
21	drug dependence	薬物依存
22	lack of appetite	食欲不振
23	food refusal; anorexia	拒食
24	overeating	過食
25	sleeplessness	不眠
26	paranoia	被害妄想
27	megalomania; grandiose delusions	誇大妄想
29	traumatic experience	心的外傷体験
30	regression	退行

Expressions　表現

① しばしば不安を感じますか。
　Do you often feel uneasy?

② とても疲れていますか。
　Do you feel very tired?

③ 物事に集中できないですか。
　Do you have difficulty concentrating?

④ ストレスがたまっていますか。
　Are you getting stressed out?

⑤ よく眠れますか。
　Can you sleep well?

⑥ 1日にどのくらいお酒を飲みますか。
　How much alcohol do you drink a day?

⑦ 気分が落ち込むのはいつですか。
　When do you feel depressed?

⑧ 高揚感(陶酔感)を感じたことはありますか。
　Have you felt euphoria?

⑨ 冷や汗をかくことがありますか。
　Do you sometimes get cold sweats?

⑩ 体重が増えるのが怖いですか。
　Are you afraid of gaining weight?

⑪ ほかの人が見えないものが見えたことがありますか。
　Have you seen things others can't see?

⑫ 相談にのってもらえる人はいますか。
　Do you have anyone you can talk to?

Maternal Nursing

母性看護

Words and Terms　基本用語

① Pregnancy：妊娠

1	**pregnancy**	妊娠
2	mother-to-be	妊婦
3	pregnancy test	妊娠検査
4	home pregnancy test	家庭用妊娠検査
5	gynecological checkup	妊婦健診
6	reproductive health	性と生殖にかかわる健康
7	intercourse	性交
8	painful intercourse	性交痛
9	artificial insemination	人工受精
10	*in vitro* fertilization [IVF]	体外受精
11	fertilized egg	受精卵
12	nidation; implantation	着床
13	ovulation	排卵
14	fertility drug	排卵誘発剤
15	〔**monthly**〕**period**	月経
16	menstruate	月経がある
17	miss one's period	月経がない
18	amenorrhea (absence of menstruation)	無月経
20	premenstrual syndrome [PMS]	月経前症候群
22	dysmenorrhea	月経困難症

1-04 Maternal Nursing

1. ☐ menorrhagia — 月経過多
2. ☐ menstrual pain (cramps) — 生理痛
3. ☐ menstrual disorder — 生理不順
4. ☐ **basal body temperature [BBT]** — **基礎体温**
6. ☐ vaginal discharge — おりもの
7. ☐ sanitary napkin (pad) — 生理用ナプキン
8. ☐ tampon — タンポン
9. ☐ contraception — 避妊
10. ☐ birth control — 〔避妊薬や避妊具を使っての〕受胎調節
12. ☐ birth control pills — 経口避妊薬(ピル)
13. ☐ intrauterine device [IUD]; coil — 避妊リング
15. ☐ contraceptive — 避妊薬, 避妊具
16. ☐ diaphragm — 避妊ペッサリー
17. ☐ elective abortion — 人工妊娠中絶
18. ☐ internal examination — 内診
19. ☐ vaginal examination — 腟内診
20. ☐ amniocentesis — 羊水穿刺
21. ☐ ultrasound — 超音波
22. ☐ nuchal translucency [NT] — 項部透過像
23. ☐ Papanicolaou smear test — パパニコロ―テスト
24. ☐ mother-to-child transmission — 母子感染

② Childbirth：出産

28. ☐ **midwife** — **助産師**
29. ☐ postpartum (maternity) blues — マタニティーブルー

1	☐ antenatal testing	出生前検査
2	☐ rectal examination	直腸診
3	☐ trimester	3カ月の期間(妊娠期間の3分の1
4		をさす)
5	☐ **normal birth**	**正常出産**
6	☐ late childbearing	高齢出産
7	☐ full term birth	正期産
8	☐ **miscarriage**	**流産**
9	☐ premature delivery	早産
10	☐ afterbirth	後産
11	☐ stillbirth	死産
12	☐ asphyxia	仮死
13	☐ fetal distress	胎児仮死
14	☐ obstetric shock	産科ショック
15	☐ perinatal period	周産期
16	☐ puerperal period	産褥期
17	☐ expected date of delivery	分娩予定日
18	☐ delivery table	分娩台
19	☐ **labor (delivery) room**	**分娩室**
20	☐ **morning sickness**	**つわり**
21	☐ amniorrhexis; water	破水
22	breaking	
23	☐ childbirth	分娩
24	☐ push	いきむ
25	☐ labor pain	陣痛
26	☐ expulsive force	娩出力
27	☐ birth canal	産道
28	☐ rotation	〔胎児の〕回旋
29	☐ face presentation	顔位(胎児顔面が先進する胎位)
30	☐ breech presentation	骨盤位(逆子の胎位)

1	☐ large baby	巨大児
2	☐ crowning	発露
3	☐ T bandage	T字帯
4	☐ Caesarean section	帝王切開
5	[C-section]	
6	☐ vacuum extraction[VE]	吸引分娩
7	☐ involution of the uterus	子宮復古
8	☐ placenta previa	前置胎盤
9	☐ epidural block	硬膜外ブロック
10	☐ engorgement	うっ積, 充血
11	☐ anemia	貧血
12	☐ tub bath	沐浴
13	☐ umbilical cord	へその緒, 臍帯
14	☐ meconium	胎便
15	☐ Eugenic Protection Act	優生保護法

③ Childcare：育児

18	☐ maternal and child health	母子保健
19	[MCH]	
20	☐ **maternal and child health**	母子手帳
21	**handbook**	
22	☐ maternal body	母体管理
23	management	
24	☐ **maternal and child health**	母子の健康
25	☐ parenting support	子育て支援
26	☐ neonatal period	新生児期
27	☐ milk secretion	乳汁分泌
28	☐ lactation	授乳
29	☐ **baby bottle**	**哺乳瓶**
30	☐ breast pump	搾乳器

1	☐ colostrum	初乳
2	☐ **weaning food**	**離乳食**
3	☐ letdown reflex	催乳反射

④ Diseases, Treatments：疾患と治療

6	☐ toxemia of pregnancy	妊娠中毒症
7	☐ pregnancy induced hypertension [PIH]	妊娠高血圧症候群
9	☐ gestational diabetes	妊娠糖尿病
10	☐ multiple pregnancy	多胎妊娠
11	☐ ectopic pregnancy	子宮外妊娠
12	☐ **infertility**	**不妊症**
13	☐ recurrent miscarriage	反復流産
14	☐ imminent abortion	切迫流産
15	☐ metrorrhagia	子宮出血
16	☐ uterine myoma	子宮筋腫
17	☐ uterine cancer	子宮がん
18	☐ **cervical cancer**	**子宮頸がん**
19	☐ genital bleeding	性器出血
20	☐ vaginitis	腟炎
21	☐ abruption of placenta	胎盤早期剥離
22	☐ subchorionic hematoma	絨毛膜下血腫
23	☐ disseminated intravascular coagulation [DIC]	播種性血管内凝固症候群
26	☐ chromosomal aberration	染色体異常
27	☐ intrauterine growth restriction [IUGR]	子宮内胎児発育遅延
29	☐ cerebral paralysis [CP]	脳性麻痺
30	☐ pre-eclampsia	子癇前症

1	☐ eclampsia	子癇
2	☐ **breast cancer**	**乳がん**
3	☐ mastitis	乳腺炎
4	☐ postnatal depression	産後うつ
5	☐ vitamin K deficiency	ビタミンK欠乏症
6	☐ cytomegalovirus infection	サイトメガロウイルス感染症
7	☐ fetal therapy	胎児治療
8-9	☐ hormone replacement therapy [HRT]	ホルモン補充療法
10	☐ episiotomy	会陰切開術
11-12	☐ dilation and curettage [D&C]	子宮内膜掻爬術

⑤ Related Terms：その他

15	☐ pelvis	骨盤
16	☐ placenta	胎盤
17	☐ vagina	腟
18	☐ uterus	子宮
19	☐ fallopian tube	卵管
20	☐ cervical canal	子宮頸管
21	☐ effacement	頸管展退度
22	☐ amniotic fluid	羊水
23	☐ embryo	胚, 胎芽
24	☐ estrogen	エストロゲン
25	☐ progesterone	プロゲステロン
26	☐ heredity	遺伝
27	☐ **menopausal disorder**	**更年期障害**
28-29	☐ simplified menopausal index [SMI]	簡易更年期指数
30	☐ **menopause**	**閉経期, 更年期**

母性看護

1. ☐ hot flash 〔閉経期の〕顔面紅潮
2. ☐ lump しこり
3. ☐ **birth rate** **出生率**
4. ☐ death rate 死亡率
5. ☐ infant mortality rate 乳児死亡率

> **column** ことわざ1
>
> ☐ 予防は治療に勝る（転ばぬ先の杖）
>   Prevention is better than cure.
> ☐ 自然は最良の医師
>   Nature is the best physician.
> ☐ 良薬は口に苦し
>   A good medicine tastes bitter.
> ☐ 死以外のすべての物事には薬がある
>   There is remedy for all things but death.
> ☐ 一日一個のりんごで医者いらず
>   An apple a day keeps the doctor away.

Expressions 表現

① Pregnancy：妊娠

①つわりがありましたか。

Have you had morning sickness?

②レモンのような酸っぱいものを食べたいと感じますか。

Do you feel like eating sour things like lemons?

③毎朝基礎体温を計ってください。

Please take your basal body temperature every morning.

④流産(中絶)をしたことがありますか。

Have you had any miscarriages (abortions)?

⑤妊娠検査は陽性(陰性)です。

Your pregnancy test is positive (negative).

⑥おめでとうございます。2週間以上も体温が高いですし、ご懐妊されたに違いありません。

Congratulations! You must be pregnant; your temperature has been high for more than two weeks.

⑦この台に上がって足を開いてください。

Please get onto the table and put your feet in the supports, bend your legs and spread your feet apart.

⑧あなたは妊娠3カ月です。

You are three months pregnant.

⑨出産予定日は10月10日です。

Your due date is October 10th.

⑩胎児の成長をエコーで調べましょう。

Let's check the development of the fetus by ultrasound.

⑪赤ちゃんの胎動を感じましたか。

Have you felt your baby's movement?

⑫腰痛やむくみがありますか。

Do you have low back pain or swelling?

⑬出産休暇がもらえますか。

Can you get maternity leave?

⑭赤ちゃんは順調に育っています。

Your baby is growing at a healthy rate.

患者さんからの表現例　妊娠

□どうにもつわりがひどいので、できればすぐに診察してもらいたいのです。
I have terrible morning sickness. If possible, I'd like to see a doctor immediately.

□どうも妊娠したらしいんです。
I think I'm pregnant.

② Childbirth：出産

①陣痛はどのくらいの間隔ですか。

How far apart are your contractions?

②陣痛誘発剤を使ってもよろしいですか。

Is it all right if we give you a drug to induce labor?

③破水しましたか。

Has your water broken?

④分娩室にお入りになって一緒にいてあげてください。
Please come to the delivery room to be with her during the birth.

⑤お子さんは逆子(順位)です。
Your baby is in the breech (head down) position.

⑥分娩は経腟分娩(帝王切開)でした。
You had a vaginal delivery (a Cesarean delivery).

③ Childcare：育児

①赤ちゃんをあやしてみてください。
Please try to comfort your baby.

②お子さんはどうしましたか。
What seems to be the problem with your child?

③お子さんの事をいつもどう呼んでいますか。
What do you usually call your child?

④ごきょうだいは何人ですか。
How many brothers or sisters does he have?

⑤これまでにひきつけを起こしたことはありますか。
Has he had any convulsive seizures?

⑥食欲はどうですか。
How is his appetite?

⑦機嫌はどうですか。
How is his mood?

⑧歯は生えてきましたか。
Is she teething?

⑨診察したいのでお子さんを抱いていてください。
Please hold your child so I can examine him.

④ Women's Health：ウィメンズヘルス

①あなたの月経周期はどのくらいですか。
How long are your menstrual cycles?

②閉経になったのはいつですか。
How old were you when you reached menopause?

③乳房の自己検診はどのくらいの頻度で行っていますか。
How often do you do breast self-examination?

④骨粗しょう症を防ぐために何をしていますか。
What are you doing to prevent osteoporosis?

⑤家庭での安全(家庭内暴力など)に関して心配がありますか。
Are you concerned for your safety at home?

患者さんからの表現例　ウィメンズヘルス

□月経があるべき日にありません。
I have missed my period.

□あと数日で月経になるのですが、生理痛がひどいのです。
In a few days my period will start, but I already have cramps.

□いつも月経が始まる前が憂鬱で仕方ないのです。
I always feel awful just before my period.

Community Health Nursing

地域看護

Words and Terms 基本用語

① Community Health Nursing：地域看護

☐ regional medical cooperation system	地域医療連携システム
☐ regional comprehensive care	地域包括ケア
☐ medical care in sparsely populated areas	過疎地域医療
☐ nursing home	養護施設, 老人ホーム
☐ **public health nurse**	**保健師**
☐ **public health center**	**保健所**
☐ clinic	診療所
☐ general〔medical〕practice	総合診療
☐ home-visit nursing station	訪問看護ステーション
☐ **visiting care**	**訪問看護**
☐ discharge support	退院支援
☐ **public health**	**公衆衛生**
☐ disease prevention	疾病予防
☐ infectious disease	感染症
☐ community medical examinations	集団検診
☐ food administration	食品管理
☐ nutritional guidance	栄養指導

	dependence on medical care	医療依存

② School Health：学校保健

	counselor	カウンセラー
	school counseling	スクールカウンセリング
	school physical examination	学校検診（健康診断）
	school nurse's office	**保健室**
	sex education	性教育
	temporary cancellation of classes	学級閉鎖
	school environmental health	学校環境衛生
	return to school	復学
	truancy	不登校
	health instruction	保健指導
	team medical care	チーム医療
	vaccination	**予防接種**
	outbreak	集団感染
	early adolescence	思春期
	precocious puberty	思春期早発症
	delayed puberty	思春期遅発症
	adolescent pregnancy	思春期妊娠
	secondary sex characteristics	第2次性徴
	growth hormone [GH]	成長ホルモン
	dysmenorrhea	月経困難症
	irregular menstruation	月経異常
	absence of menstruation	無月経

1	☐ sexually transmitted disease [STD]	性感染症
3	☐ family background	家庭環境
4	☐ growth curve	成長曲線
5	☐ stadiometer	身長計
6	☐ weight scale	体重計
7	☐ eye test	視力検査
8	☐ hearing test	聴力検査
9	☐ body mass index [BMI]	体格指数
10	☐ body fat percentage	体脂肪率
11	☐ emaciation	るいそう
12	☐ growth disorder	成長障害

③ Stressful Life Events：ストレスになる出来事

15	☐ child abuse	児童虐待
16	☐ family discord	家庭不和
17	☐ family breakdown	家庭崩壊
18	☐ parents' divorce	親の離婚
19	☐ breakup of a family	家庭の崩壊
20	☐ underachiever	落ちこぼれ
21	☐ **bullying**	いじめ
22	☐ outcast	のけ者
23	☐ failure in the entrance examination	受験の失敗
25	☐ to be held back; repeat a grade in school	留年
27	☐ job shortage	就職難
28	☐ domestic violence	ドメスティックバイオレンス, 家庭内暴力

1	☐ trouble between one's wife and one's mother	嫁姑問題
3	☐ entrance	入学
4	☐ transfer of schools	転校
5	☐ graduation	卒業
6	☐ suspension from school	出席停止

④ Related Terms：その他

9	**child guidance center**	**児童相談所**
10	☐ child-rearing allowance	児童扶養手当
11	**child welfare**	**児童福祉**
12	☐ Children's Charter	児童憲章
13	**children's home**	**児童養護施設**
14	☐ temporary childcare services; foster care	一時的保育サービス
16	☐ three-year-old infant check-up	3歳児健診
18	☐ home for fatherless families	母子寮
20	☐ foster parent	里親
21	☐ family policy	家庭の方針
22	☐ dietary guidelines	食事の指針

Expressions 表現

① いじめを受けたことはありますか。
Have you experienced bullying?

② 勉強はどうですか。
How is your studying going?

③ 月経は規則的にありますか。
Do you have a regular menstrual period?

④ ダイエットをしていますか。
Are you on a diet?

⑤ もっと休んでください。
You need more rest.

⑥ 泣いてもいいですよ。
It's OK to cry.

⑦ 健康診断の結果は2週間後にわかります。
You'll have the results of the checkup in two weeks.

⑧ 医師に診てもらったほうがいいでしょう。
You had better see a doctor.

⑨ カウンセラーに相談したほうがいいでしょう。
You had better consult a counselor.

⑩ お母さんに来てもらうよう頼みました。
I asked your mother to come.

⑪ 救急車を呼びます。
I'll call an ambulance.

⑫ インフルエンザが治るまで学校は休んでください。
Please stay at home until you recover from the flu.

Geriatric Nursing
老年看護

Words and Terms 基本用語

① General Terms：一般用語

1. ☐ aging society — 高齢化社会
2. ☐ super-aged society — 超高齢社会
3. ☐ welfare — 福祉
4. ☐ medical insurance system for the elderly aged 75 or over — 後期高齢者医療制度
5. ☐ Health and Medical Service Act for the Aged — 老人保健法
6. ☐ comprehensive geriatric assessment — 高齢者総合機能評価
7. ☐ healthy life expectancy — 健康寿命
8. ☐ terminal care — 〔終末期〕ターミナルケア
9. ☐ healthcare facility for the elderly — 老人保健施設
10. ☐ special nursing home — 特別養護老人ホーム
11. ☐ senile dementia center — 老人性痴呆疾患センター
12. ☐ senior citizens' club — 老人クラブ
13. ☐ group home — グループホーム
14. ☐ **daily activity center for elderly** — デイケア
15. ☐ day service — デイサービス
16. ☐ short stay — ショートステイ

1	degree of aging	老化度
2	**bedridden elderly**	**寝たきり老人**
3-5	campaign to prevent from becoming bedridden	寝たきり老人ゼロ作戦
6-7	geriatric depression scale [GDS]	老年期うつ尺度
8	fall risk evaluation	転倒リスク評価
9	health problem	健康障害
10	position change	体位交換
11	suction	吸痰
12	endstage	末期
13	loitering	徘徊
14	incontinence	失禁
15	diaper	おむつ
16	fall prevention	転倒防止
17	requiring care	要介護
18	cancer nursing	がん看護
19	deathwatch	看取り
20	palliative care	緩和ケア

② Diseases, Treatments：疾患と治療

23	cognitive function decline	認知機能低下
24	**dementia**	**認知症**
25	vascular dementia	血管性認知症
26-27	dementia with Lewy bodies [DLB]	レビー小体型認知症
28	frontotemporal dementia	前頭側頭型認知症
29	senile dementia	老人性認知症
30	Alzheimer's disease	アルツハイマー病

老年看護

1. ☐ Parkinson's disease — パーキンソン病
2. ☐ mild cognitive impairment [MCI] — 軽度認知障害
3. ☐ behavioral and psychological symptoms of dementia [BPSD] — 認知症の行動・心理症状
4. ☐ core symptom — 中核症状
5. ☐ osteoporosis — 骨粗鬆症
6. ☐ malnutrition — 低栄養
7. ☐ sarcopenia — 筋肉減少症(サルコペニア)
8. ☐ swallowing difficulty — 嚥下障害
9. ☐ aspiration — 誤嚥
10. ☐ senile pneumonia — 高齢者肺炎
11. ☐ geriatric syndrome — 老年症候群
12. ☐ disuse syndrome — 廃用症候群

③ Nursing Concerns：患者さんへの配慮

- ☐ listening — 傾聴
- ☐ **supportive presence** — 共にいること
- ☐ dignity — 尊厳
- ☐ **psychological care** — 心のケア
- ☐ grief care — 悲嘆ケア
- ☐ purpose in life — 生きがい
- ☐ reason for being; the purpose of one's existence — 存在価値
- ☐ self-respect — 自尊心
- ☐ self-esteem — 自己尊重
- ☐ sense of security — 安心感
- ☐ sedation — 鎮静

- change of pace　　　　気分転換

④ Terminal Care and Death：終末期ケアと死

- care of a family member　　家族の介護
- incurable disease　　不治の病
- terminal stage　　末期
- hospice　　ホスピス
- **alleviation**　　**緩和**
- bedsore　　床ずれ
- loneliness　　孤独感
- faint　　気絶
- kin / next of kin　　親族／最近親者
- pass away　　亡くなる
- death of a family member　　家族の死
- death of a close relative　　近親者の死
- death of one's spouse　　配偶者の死
- suicide / homicide; murder　　自殺／殺人
- spirit; soul　　魂
- euthanasia　　安楽死
- mercy killing　　慈悲殺
- death with dignity　　尊厳死
- natural death　　自然死
- brain death　　脳死
- accidental death　　事故死
- sudden death　　突然死
- cardiac death　　心臓死
- death from suffocation / starvation　　窒息死／餓死
- advance directive　　事前指示〔書〕

1	☐ do not resuscitate [DNR]	蘇生処置を拒絶すること
2	☐ **death education**	デス・エデュケーション, 死への準備教育
4	☐ death certificate	死亡証明書, 死亡診断書
5	☐ death instinct	死の本能
6	☐ death rattle	死前喘鳴
7	☐ deathwatch	死の看取り
8	☐ death and dying	死と臨終
9	☐ death struggle (agony)	死のもがき
10	☐ **five stages of dying**	死にゆく過程の5段階
11	**1. denial**	拒否
12	**2. anger**	怒り
13	**3. bargaining**	取り引き
14	**4. depression**	抑うつ
15	**5. acceptance**	受容
16	☐ sense of defeat	敗北感
17	☐ denial	否認
18	☐ loss	喪失感
19	☐ burnout	極度の疲労, 燃え尽き症候群
20	☐ grief	悲嘆
21	☐ sadness	悲しみ
22	☐ despair	絶望
23	☐ lethargy	無気力
24	☐ disinterest	無関心
25	☐ meaninglessness	無意味さ
26	☐ distrust	不信
27	☐ self-disgust	自己嫌悪
28	☐ self-denial	自己否定
29	☐ palliative care (treatment)	緩和ケア(治療)
30	☐ palliation	一時的緩和(軽減)

1	☐ painkiller	鎮痛剤
2	☐ spiritual well-being	霊的安寧
3	☐ pain management	疼痛処理
4	☐ comfort measures	安楽のケア
5	☐ respite care	レスパイトケア(一時的対応)
6	☐ funeral arrangements	葬式の準備(手配)
7,8	☐ withdrawal of life support system (machinery)	生命維持装置の停止
9	☐ autopsy	検死
10	☐ victim	犠牲者
11	☐ casualty	死傷者
12	☐ rigor mortis	死後硬直
13	☐ death spots	死斑

---

column　心のケア

患者さんに対して，検査・治療などを最適な方法で行うことは当然ですが，同時に「心のケア」が，高齢者には特に必要です。高齢になると若い頃の「楽しみ」「希望」が徐々に減ってきますが，高齢者の「楽しみ」「希望」を一緒に見つけることも看護のプロとして大変重要です。患者さんのQOLを高める努力を最期の瞬間まで怠らないでください。

☐人生とはただ生きることでなく楽しむことである。
　Life consists not in breathing but in enjoying life.
☐生命あるかぎり希望あり
　While there is life, there is hope.
☐死以外のすべての物事には薬がある
　There is remedy for all things but death.

老年看護

Expressions　表現

①おつらいでしょう。何かお手伝いできますか。
I am sure this must be difficult for you. How can I help you?

②残念なお知らせがあるのです。
I'm afraid the news is not good.

③おそばにおりますから安らかにお眠りください。
Rest while we care for you.

④おそばにいますから何でも話してください。
I'm here to listen to you.

⑤楽になられますようにおそばにいますよ。
I'm here to make you comfortable.

⑥～さんとお二人だけの方がよろしいですか？
Do you wish to be alone with... ?

⑦ご家族の方に連絡しましょうか。
Do you want us to notify any of your family?

⑧すぐお出でいただけますか。お母様の容態が急変いたしました。
Can you come right away? Your mother's condition has changed suddenly.

⑨ご家族の皆様にはご連絡なさいましたか。
Have you notified all of her family members?

⑩お父様は心停止されました。残念です。出来るだけのことをいたしましたが、力が及びませんでした。
Your father went into cardiac arrest. I'm sorry. We did everything we could, but we weren't able to revive him.

⑪お気の毒に思います。
I'm sorry. / I am sad for you.

⑫心からお悔やみ申し上げます。
　Please accept my deepest sympathy (condolence).
⑬お父様の清拭のお手伝いをなさいますか。
　Would you like to help us bathe your father?

患者さんからの表現例　終末期ケア

□楽になるようにしてくださいませんか。
　Could you make me comfortable, please?
□しばらくそばにいてくださいませんか。
　Would you be with me for a while?
□1人にしてくれませんか。
　You can leave now. I'd like to be alone.

Home Care Nursing
在宅看護

Words and Terms 基本用語

1. ☐ family doctor — かかりつけ医
2. ☐ **care manager** — **ケアマネージャー**
3. ☐ caseworker — ケースワーカー
4. ☐ 〔certified〕caregiver — 〔認定〕ケアワーカー
5. ☐ medical social worker — 医療ソーシャルワーカー
6. ☐ home-care worker — ホームヘルパー
7. ☐ helper — ヘルパー
8. ☐ key person — キーパーソン
9. ☐ interprofessional collaboration — 専門職種間連携
11. ☐ national health insurance — 国民健康保険
12. ☐ medical insurance system — 医療保険制度
13. ☐ **care insurance** — **介護保険**
14. ☐ medical insurance system for the elderly aged 75 or over — 後期高齢者医療制度
17. ☐ **care support** — **介護支援**
18. ☐ **home-visit care** — **訪問介護**
19. ☐ home palliative treatment — 在宅緩和医療
20. ☐ home welfare measures — 在宅福祉対策
21. ☐ home-care management — 居宅療養管理指導
22. ☐ home-visit dietary instruction — 訪問栄養食事指導

1	☐ **care plan**	ケアプラン
2	☐ home care	在宅ケア
3	☐ home-delivery service	宅配サービス
4	☐ self-care	セルフケア
5	☐ hotline	ホットライン
6	☐ nursing care benefit	介護給付
7	☐ training benefit	訓練等給付
8	☐ home-care support center	在宅介護支援センター
9	☐ **home nursing station**	**訪問看護ステーション**
10	☐ home-care management fee	在宅療養指導管理料
12	☐ respite care	レスパイトケア(一時的休息)
13	☐ locomotive syndrome	ロコモティブシンドローム
14	☐ respiratory management	呼吸管理
15	☐ home mechanical ventilation [HMV]	在宅人工呼吸療法
17	☐ suction	吸痰
18	☐ pulse oxymeter	パルスオキシメーター
19	☐ self-injection	自己注射
20	☐ insulin	インスリン
21	☐ home parenteral nutrition [HPN]	在宅中心静脈栄養
23	☐ social rehabilitation	社会復帰
24	☐ care equipment	介護機器
25	☐ home monitoring system	在宅モニタリングシステム
26	☐ portable transfusion system	携帯用輸液システム
28	☐ home oxygen therapy [HOT]	在宅酸素療法
30	☐ portable oxygen bottle	携帯酸素ボンベ

Expressions 表現

①はじめまして。
Nice to meet you.

②六本木訪問看護ステーションから参りました山本愛です。
I am Ai Yamamoto, a nurse from Roppongi Visiting Nursing Station.

③訪問看護サービスの内容を確認させていただきます。
I would like to go over the services of this homevisiting nursing care service.

④訪問看護師にどういう事をして欲しいですか。
What would you like a visiting nurse to do for you?

⑤健康上の問題を教えてください。
Please describe your health problem.

⑥ホームヘルパーさんが必要ですか。
Do you need a home-care worker?

⑦私は週に2回,月曜日と木曜日に参ります。
I will visit you twice a week, on Mondays and Thursdays.

⑧具合が悪くなったらいつでも知らせてください。電話番号は×××-××××-××××です。
Please let us know whenever you feel ill. Our telephone number is ×××-××××-××××.

⑨私が訪問するときは毎回血圧と体温を測らせていただきます。
I will take your blood pressure and temperature at every visit.

⑩検査を受けられた方がいいと思います。
Some tests may be needed.

⑪近くの六本木病院に行かれてはどうでしょうか。
How about going to Roppongi Hospital near here?

⑫サービス料金についてはパンフレットをご覧ください。
Please refer to the pamphlet about the cost for service.

⑬健康保険証はおもちですか。
Do you have a health insurance card?

⑭日常生活について教えてください。
Please tell me about your daily life.

⑮朝食は何を召し上がりましたか。
What did you have for breakfast?

⑯おうちに帰られてからお元気になられたと思いますよ。
I think you have gotten better since you came home.

⑰今日具合はいかがですか。
How are you feeling today?

⑱医師に往診してもらうように頼みます。
I will ask a doctor to visit you.

⑲緊急の場合どなたに連絡すればいいですか。
Whom should I contact in an emergency?

⑳私達のケアに満足いただいていますか。
Are you satisfied with our care?

㉑ご家族のケアで何かお困りのことがありますか。
Are you experiencing difficulties in caring for your family?

㉒介護は疲れるものですが, あなたはいかがですか?
Being a caregiver can be tiring. How are you doing?

在宅看護

 患者さんからの表現例 **訪問看護**

□訪問看護に来ていただきありがとうございます。
Thank you for visiting me for nursing care.

□身体を動かすのを手伝ってください。
I would like you to help me change position.

□お薬の飲み方がわからなくなったので、もう一度おさらいさせてください。
I am confused about medications. Please review them with me.

□具合が悪いときはどなたに連絡すればいいですか。
Whom should I contact if I get worse (have a problem)?

□真夜中でも連絡していいですか。
Can I contact you even during the night?

□熱が出たらどうすればいいですか。
What shall I do if I have a fever?

□家族が留守のときは頻繁に来ていただけませんか。
Will you visit me more frequently when my family members are away?

□今度はいつ来てもらえますか。
When will you visit me next?

□お支払いはどうすればよいですか。
What should I do about the payment?

□病院に連れていってもらえますか。
Will you take me to the hospital?

□診察を受けにどこに行けばいいでしょうか。
Where should I go to see a doctor?

Fundamental Nursing
基礎看護

Words and Terms　基本用語

① Insurance and Health Care Financing：健康保険関連用語

1. ☐ health care benefit〔coverage〕　〔健康〕保険給付
2. **☐ health insurance**　**健康保険**
3. ☐ eligibility　適格性
4. ☐ patient's copayment system　患者一部負担制度
5. ☐ public funding　公的資金
6. ☐ medical assistance program　医療援助プログラム
7. ☐ medical care benefit　医療給付
8. ☐ medical care plan　医療計画
9. **☐ universal health insurance coverage**　**国民皆保険制度**
10. ☐ drug tariff　薬価基準
11. ☐ employees' pension　厚生年金

② Public Health：公衆衛生

(a) General Terms：一般用語

- ☐ World Health Organization〔WHO〕　世界保健機関

基礎看護

1. **Ministry of Health, Labour and Welfare** — 厚生労働省
2. Council on Public Health — 公衆衛生審議会
3. national hospital organization — 国立病院機構
4. national hospital — 国立病院
5. general hospital — 総合病院
6. medical center — 医療センター
7. public health center — 保健所
8. clinic — 診療所
9. mental health center — 精神保健センター
10. municipal health center — 市町村保健センター
11. welfare commissioner — 民生委員
12. regional health and medical care plan — 地域保健医療計画
13. bone-marrow bank — 骨髄バンク
14. countermeasure against cancer — がん対策
15. Human Genome Project [HGP] — ヒトゲノムプロジェクト
16. triage — 治療優先順位の選別
17. **primary care** — プライマリーケア
18. alternative healthcare practitioner — 代替医療プラクティショナー
19. outpatient therapy — 外来治療
20. blood donation — 献血
21. blood product — 血液製剤
22. clinical laboratory — 衛生検査所
23. emergency medical technician [EMT] — 救急救命士

PART1 主な看護分野の基本用語と表現

1	emergency care system	救急医療システム
2	**nurse's license**	**看護師免許**
3	projection of supply and demand for nursing personnel	看護職員需給見通し
6	Act on Public Health Nurses, Midwives and Nurses	保健師助産師看護師法
9	organ donation	臓器提供
10	Organ Transplant Law	臓器移植法
11	Japan Medical Association [JMA]	日本医師会
13	Medical Practitioners' Act	医師法
14	Japanese Red Cross Society	日本赤十字社
16	social welfare	社会福祉
17	welfare state	福祉国家
18	welfare facility of social insurance	社会保険の福祉施設
20	**health promotion**	**健康増進**
21	Health Promotion Act	健康増進法
22	physically disabled person	身体障害者
24	Basic Disability Pension	障害基礎年金
25	Association for Welfare of the Mentally and Physically Disabled	心身障害者福祉協会
28	human resource agency for welfare services	福祉人材バンク

1	☐ **disaster**	災害
2	☐ disaster countermeasure	災害対策
3	☐ emergency shelter	緊急避難所
4	☐ emergency evacuation route	緊急避難経路
6	☐ National Disaster Act	災害救助法

(b) Epidemiology：疫学

8	☐ **public health**	**公衆衛生**
9	☐ sanitation inspector	衛生検査官
10	☐ pollution	公害, 汚染
11	☐ environmental sanitation	環境衛生
12	☐ contagious; infectious	感染性の
13	☐ contaminated	〔土壌, 水質などが〕汚染された
14	☐ infectious medical waste	感染性医療廃棄物
15	☐ Immunization Law	予防接種法
16	☐ surveillance system for tuberculosis and infectious diseases	結核・感染症サーベイランスシステム
19	☐ **public health center**	**保健所**
20	☐ **public health nurse**	**保健師**
21	☐ food sanitation	食品衛生
22	☐ food handlers	食品取扱業者
23	☐ health inspector	衛生指導員
24	☐ hygiene	衛生学
25	☐ parasite	寄生虫
26	☐ dioxin	ダイオキシン
27	☐ measures for infectious disease control	伝染病対策
29	☐ quarantine	検疫, 隔離

1-2	☐ Infectious Disease Prevention Act	伝染病予防法
3	☐ AIDS Prevention Law	エイズ予防法
4	☐ Global Program on AIDS	エイズ対策特別計画
5	☐ Public Health Service Act	公衆衛生法
6	☐ poison control center	中毒事故管理センター
7	☐ sewage treatment facility	下水処理施設
8	☐ water utility	水道施設
9	☐ air quality index	大気質指数
10	☐ **average life expectancy**	平均寿命
11	☐ life table	生命表
12	☐ mean	平均値
13	☐ morbidity	病的状態, 罹病率
14	☐ patient survey	患者調査
15	☐ incidence rate	発生率
16	☐ **prevalence rate**	**罹患率**
17	☐ perinatal mortality rate	周産期死亡率
18	☐ sample	サンプル, 試料, 標本
19	☐ **population**	**人口**
20	☐ vital statistics	人口動態統計
21	☐ census	人口調査
22	☐ divorce rate	離婚率
23	☐ marriage rate	婚姻率
24	☐ information systems	情報システム

③ Nursing Care Planning 看護計画関連用語

1. ☐ nursing interview [NI] — 看護面接
2. ☐ nursing diagnosis [ND] — 看護診断
3. ☐ **nursing process** — **看護過程**
4.   **1. assessment** — アセスメント
5.   **2. planning** — 計画
6.   **3. implementation** — 実施
7.   **4. evaluation** — 評価
8. ☐ SOAP charting — 問題志向型記録の形式
9.   1. subjective data [S] — 主観的所見
10.   2. objective data [O] — 客観的所見
11.   3. assessment [A] — アセスメント
12.   4. plan [P] — 計画
13. ☐ nursing care plan — 看護計画
14. ☐ diagnostic scheme — 診断計画
15. ☐ therapeutic plan — 治療計画
16. ☐ educational plan — 教育計画
17. ☐ progress notes — 経過記録
18. ☐ quality control [QC] — 〔看護の〕質の管理
19. ☐ patient-nurse interaction — 患者−看護師関係
20. ☐ telephone order — 電話指示
21. ☐ written order — 記述された指示
22. ☐ primary nursing — プライマリーナーシング
23. ☐ **quality of life [QOL]** — **生活の質**
24. ☐ diagnosis related group [DRG] — 疾病関連群
26. ☐ critical path method [CPM] — クリティカル・パス法

1-2	**problem-based learning [PBL]**	問題解決型教育法
3-5	Cumulative Index for Nursing and Allied Health Literature [CINAHL]	看護データベース
6-7	evidence-based medicine [EBM]	根拠に基づく医療
8-9	evidence-based healthcare [EBHC]	根拠に基づく医療
10-11	**evidence-based nursing [EBN]**	根拠に基づく看護
12-13	**Japanese Nursing Association [JNA]**	日本看護協会
14-15	**International Council of Nurses [ICN]**	国際看護師協会
16	nursing audit committee	看護監査委員会

④ Nursing Specialties 看護専門分野

19	introduction to nursing	看護学概論
20	fundamental nursing	基礎看護〔学〕
21-22	community health nursing	地域看護〔学〕
23	midwifery	助産学
24	psychiatric nursing	精神看護〔学〕
25	pediatric nursing	小児看護〔学〕
26	adult nursing	成人看護〔学〕
27	geriatric nursing	老人看護〔学〕
28	nursing informatics	看護情報学
29	nursing theory	看護理論
30	nursing science	看護科学

基礎看護

1	nursing sociology	看護社会学
2	medical sociology	医療社会学
3	**nursing research**	**看護研究**
4	nursing research methodology	看護研究法
6	nursing education	看護教育〔学〕
7	maternal nursing	母性看護
8	maternal-child nursing	母子看護
9	family nursing	家族看護
10	acute-care nursing	急性期看護
11	surgical nursing	手術看護
12	operating room nursing	手術室看護
13	critical care nursing	集中治療看護
14	cancer nursing; oncology nursing	がん看護
16	infection control nursing	感染管理看護
17	anesthesia nursing	麻酔看護
18	occupational health nursing	職業保健
20	primary health care nursing	プライマリーケア・ナーシング
22	school health	学校保健
23	emergency nursing	救急看護
24	visiting nursing	訪問看護
25	home care nursing	在宅看護
26	liaison nursing	リエゾン看護
27	psychiatric-liaison nursing	精神科リエゾン看護
29	nursing administration	看護管理

1. ☐ nursing service delivery system — 看護提供システム
2. ☐ clinical nursing — 臨床看護
3. ☐ nursing practice — 看護実習
4. ☐ nursing skills; nursing arts — 看護技術
5. ☐ nursing ethics — 看護倫理
6. ☐ health and welfare policy — 保健福祉政策
7. ☐ women's health — ウィメンズヘルス

---

column 看護雑誌の略称

略称	正式名称
J. Adv. Nurs.	= Journal of Advanced Nursing
J. Nurs. Staff Dev.	= Journal of Nursing Staff Development
Nurs. Health Sci.	= Nursing & Health Science
Aust. J. Adv. Nur.	= Australian Journal of Advanced Nursing
Nurs. Stand.	= Nursing Standard
Hospice J.	= Hospice Journal
Int. J. Nurs. Stud.	= International Journal of Nursing Studies
Patient Educ. Couns.	= Patient Education Counseling
Nurs. Times	= Nursing Times
J. Clin. Nurs.	= Journal of Clinical Nursing
J. Nurs. Admin.	= Journal of Nursing Administration

Expressions　表現

①健康保険をお持ちですか。
Do you have any health insurance?

②健康保険が日本の診察でも使えるかご確認ください。
Please check if your health insurance covers consultations in Japan.

③息子さんは臓器提供者カード（ドナーカード）にサインされていますか。
Has your son signed an organ-donor card?

④緊急時にはこの避難経路を進んでください。
Please follow the emergency escape route in an emergency.

⑤来週緊急避難訓練をします。
We'll have an emergency evacuation drill next week.

⑥私がプライマリーナースです。
I'm your primary nurse.

⑦私がケアプラン（看護計画）を担当します。
I'm in charge of your nursing care plan.

⑧こちらがケアプランです。
Here is the care plan for you.

⑨ケアプランの変更をご希望ですか。
Would you like to change the care plan?

⑩代替医療を受けられますか。
Will you get any alternative treatment?

⑪代替医療についてご説明します。
I'll explain alternative treatment to you.

PART 2

病棟で使われる基本用語と表現

Facility

病院施設

Words and Terms　基本用語

① Ward, Unit：病棟

1. ☐ general ward — 一般病棟
2. ☐ **emergency ward** — **救急病棟**
3. ☐ contagious disease ward — 伝染病棟
4. ☐ hospital room — 病室
5. ☐ private room — 個室
6. ☐ **nurses' station** — **ナースステーション**
7. ☐ restroom — 洗面所
8. ☐ bathroom — 風呂場
9. ☐ shower room — シャワー室
10. ☐ **lavatory; toilet; restroom** — **トイレ**
11. ☐ laundry room — 洗濯室
12. ☐ coin laundry — コインランドリー
13. ☐ **consultation room** — **診察室**
14. ☐ treatment room — 処置室
15. ☐ patients' lounge — 談話室
16. ☐ **emergency exit** — **非常口**
17. ☐ smoke alarm — 火災報知機
18. ☐ play room — プレイルーム（小児科病棟内）
19. ☐ vending machine — 自動販売機
20. ☐ fire extinguisher — 消火器
21. ☐ **operating room [OR]; surgical theater** — **手術室**

1	☐ recovery room	回復室
2	☐ **intensive care unit [ICU]**	集中治療室
3	☐ coronary care unit [CCU]	冠状動脈疾患集中治療室
4	☐ perinatal center	周産期センター
5	☐ delivery room	分娩室
6	☐ nursery	新生児室
7	☐ **rehabilitation center**	リハビリテーションセンター
8	☐ radiography (X-ray) department	放射線科
10	☐ laboratory	検査室
11	☐ blood lab	採血室
12	☐ physiological lab department	生理機能検査室
14	☐ endoscopy department	内視鏡検査室

② Outpatient Department：外来

17	☐ general reception	総合受付
18	☐ information counter	案内係
19	☐ registration	新患受付
20	☐ admission office	入院受付
21	☐ outpatient window	外来窓口
22	☐ **cashier**	会計窓口
23	☐ lobby	ロビー
24	☐ hall	廊下
25	☐ stairs	階段
26	☐ elevator	エレベーター
27	☐ waiting room (area)	待合室
28	☐ **pharmacy**	薬局
29	☐ **ambulance**	救急車

③ Patient's Room：病室

- [ ] window shade　　　　　　　ブラインド
- [ ] bedding　　　　　　　　　　寝具一式
- [ ] bedside table　　　　　　　床頭台
- [ ] bedrail　　　　　　　　　　ベッド柵, ベッドレール
- [ ] [bed] sheet　　　　　　　　シーツ
- [ ] bidet　　　　　　　　　　　お尻洗浄器
- [ ] **call button; call bell**　　　**ナースコール**
- [ ] locker　　　　　　　　　　　ロッカー
- [ ] electric blanket　　　　　　電気毛布
- [ ] foot rail　　　　　　　　　　足下のベッド柵, フットレール
- [ ] **hospital gown**　　　　　　**病衣**
- [ ] mattress　　　　　　　　　マットレス
- [ ] over the bed table　　　　　オーバーベッドテーブル
- [ ] **oxygen outlet**　　　　　　**酸素プラグ差込口**
- [ ] quilt; duvet; comforter　　　ふとん
- [ ] bathrobe　　　　　　　　　バスローブ
- [ ] refrigerator　　　　　　　　冷蔵庫
- [ ] wastebasket; rubbish bin　　ゴミ箱
- [ ] basket　　　　　　　　　　〔衣類の〕かご

④ Other Areas：その他のエリア

- [ ] cafeteria; dining room　　　食堂
- [ ] café　　　　　　　　　　　喫茶室
- [ ] flower shop　　　　　　　　花屋
- [ ] store　　　　　　　　　　　売店
- [ ] barbershop　　　　　　　　理髪店
- [ ] taxi stand　　　　　　　　　タクシー乗り場
- [ ] mortuary　　　　　　　　　霊安室

⑤ Nursing Supplies：看護用品

- [ ] absorbent cotton; cotton balls 脱脂綿
- [ ] **adhesive bandage; adhesive tape** **絆創膏**
- [ ] tampon タンポン, 綿球
- [ ] cotton swab; Q-tip 綿棒
- [ ] gauze ガーゼ
- [ ] antiseptic solution 消毒液
- [ ] **disinfectant cotton** **消毒綿**
- [ ] disinfectant 殺菌(消毒)剤
- [ ] **bandage; dressing** **包帯**
- [ ] Band-Aid バンドエイド(救急絆創膏の商標)
- [ ] distilled water 蒸留水
- [ ] lukewarm water ぬるま湯
- [ ] boiling water 熱湯
- [ ] chest binder 胸帯
- [ ] abdominal binder 腹帯
- [ ] **eye patch** **眼帯**
- [ ] filter paper 濾紙
- [ ] oiled paper 油紙
- [ ] finger cot 指サック
- [ ] plastic pad ケリーパッド
- [ ] splash guard 防水シート
- [ ] **surgical gown (cap; mask)** 手術用着衣(帽子, マスク)
- [ ] **latex gloves** **ラテックス手袋**
- [ ] rubber glove (sheet; tube) ゴム製手袋(シート, チューブ)

1	☐ lancet	ランセット
2	☐ small forceps	ピンセット
3	☐ forceps	鉗子
4	☐ clamp	クランプ, 鉗子
5	☐ scalpel	外科用メス
6	☐ **endoscope**	**内視鏡**
7	☐ needle〔for injection〕	注射針
8	☐ syringe	注射器, 注入器
9	☐ oxygen mask	酸素マスク
10	☐ ice pack (pillow)	氷嚢, 氷枕
11	☐ hot-water bottle	湯たんぽ
12	☐ pressure bandage	圧迫帯
13	(dressing)	
14	☐ sling	吊り包帯, 三角巾
15	☐ **disposable diaper**	**紙オムツ**
16	☐ Petri dish	〔蓋付きの〕シャーレ, ペトリ皿
17	☐ **test tube**	**試験管**
18	☐ tongue depressor	舌圧子
19	☐ artificial arm (hand; leg)	義手, 義足
20	☐ bifocals	遠近両用眼鏡
21	☐ brace	〔整形外科的〕装具
22	☐ crown	歯冠
23	☐ dentures	総入れ歯
24	☐ false (artificial) teeth	入れ歯, 義歯
25	☐ prosthesis	人工器官, 人工装具 (義眼, 義足
26		など)
27	☐ hearing aid	補聴器

⑥ Equipment for Care：看護機器

☐ **medical supplies**	処置用具
☐ armrest	〔注射時に腕の下に置く〕小枕
☐ aspirator	吸引器
☐ bed-pan	差込み便器
☐ blood pressure gauge; sphygmomanometer	血圧計
☐ vacuum extraction tube system	真空採血管
☐ blood sample holder	採血用ホルダー
☐ cuff	カフ（血圧計の加圧帯）
☐ tourniquet	止血帯,圧迫帯
☐ compressed air outlet	圧縮空気差込プラグ
☐ crutch (crutches)	松葉杖
☐ corset	コルセット
☐ cast	ギプス
☐ **stick; cane**	**杖**
☐ splint	副木
☐ drain tube	排水チューブ
☐ defibrillator	除細動器
☐ **infectious waste bin**	**危険物廃棄ボックス**
☐ inhaler	吸入器
☐ irrigator	洗浄器,イリガトール
☐ intravenous injection [IV] pole	点滴用ポール
☐ leg-rest; footrest	レッグレスト,脚のせ
☐ walker〔with brakes〕	〔ブレーキ付き〕歩行器
☐ **wheelchair[WC]**	**車椅子**
☐ **stretcher; gurney**	**担架,ストレッチャー**

2-01 Facility

1. ☐ **medication (IV) cart** — 与薬(点滴)カート
2. ☐ crash cart — クラッシュカート, 救急ワゴン
3. ☐ dressing cart — 包帯交換ワゴン, 包交車
4. ☐ shampoo cart — 洗髪車
5. ☐ monitor — 監視装置
6. ☐ nebulizer — 噴霧器
7. ☐ operating table — 手術台
8. ☐ oxygen tank — 酸素タンク
9. ☐ **ventilator** — **人工呼吸器**
10. ☐ respirator — 人口呼吸装置
11. ☐ **suction machine / outlet** — **吸引器／差込プラグ**
12. ☐ steam inhaler — 蒸気吸入器
13. ☐ ring shaped cushion — 円座
14. ☐ gastric (stomach) tube — 胃管
15. ☐ naso-gastric tube — 経鼻胃管
16. ☐ **stethoscope** — **聴診器**
17. ☐ **thermometer** — **体温計**
18. ☐ truss — ヘルニアバンド, 脱腸帯
19. ☐ treatment table — 処置台
20. ☐ tube stand — 検体立て
21. ☐ enema; syringe — 浣腸〔器〕
22. ☐ **urinal** — **蓄尿器**
23. ☐ **urine bottle** — **採尿器, しびん**
24. ☐ portable toilet; commode — ポータブルトイレ
25. ☐ 〔emesis〕 basin — 嘔吐盆
26. ☐ spittoon — 痰壺
27. ☐ measuring cup (spoon; tape) — 計量カップ(計量スプーン, メジャー)
29. ☐ tray — トレイ

病院施設

1. ☐ stadiometer — 身長計
2. ☐ weight scale — 体重計
3. ☐ **scale; balance** — **はかり**
4. ☐ pitcher — 水差し
5. ☐ filter — 濾過器
6. ☐ flashlight — 懐中電灯
7. ☐ foot-bath tub — 足浴用洗面器
8. ☐ head mirror — 額帯鏡

column °F/°C換算

華氏（°F）と摂氏（°C）の換算方法
°F ＝ °C × 9/5 ＋ 32°　　°C ＝（°F-32）× 5/9

華氏 (Fahrenheit)	摂氏 (Centigrade)
104	40.0
103	39.4
102	38.9
101	38.3
100	37.8
99	37.2
98	36.7
97	36.1

Expressions 表現

① 入院準備：Preparation for Hospitalization

①検査(手術)のために入院する必要があります。
You need to be hospitalized for some tests (an operation).

②ベッドが空き次第, 入院になります。
You will be called just as soon as a bed becomes available.

③ご家族の連絡先を教えてください。
Please leave the contact address of your family.

患者さんからの表現例　入院準備

☐ 入院するときに何を準備したらいいか教えてください。
Please tell me what I should prepare for hospitalization.

☐ 自分のパジャマとパソコンを持ち込んでもいいですか。
Can I bring my pajamas and computer to the hospital?

☐ この病院で使用する携帯電話とテレビを借りることができますか。
Can I borrow a cell phone and TV here at the hospital?

☐ 手術のあと何日くらいの入院が必要ですか。
How many days do I have to stay in the hospital after the surgery?

② 入院生活：Life in Hospital

①どのメニューにしますか。
What would you like to eat?

②日本食をお食べになりますか。
Do you eat Japanese food?

③食事は流動食(普通食)になります。
You will have a liquid (normal) diet.

④食器を下げてもよろしいですか。
May I clear away the dishes?

⑤食事は配膳車に戻してください。
Please return the dishes to the waiting cart.

⑥間食をしないでください。
Please don't eat between meals.

⑦面会時間は午後3時から7時までです。
Visiting hours are from 3:00 p.m. to 7:00 p.m.

⑧ご用があるときはこのボタンを押してください。
Please push this button if you need any help.

⑨先生の回診は午前11時です。
The doctor makes her (his) rounds at 11:00 a.m.

⑩シーツを直して枕をふわりとしましょう。
Let me make the bed and fluff the pillow.

⑪～さんが面会に来られています。
Ms. (Mr.)... has come to visit you.

⑫看護学生と研修医が訓練にやって来るでしょう。
Student nurses and residents will visit you for their training.

患者さんからの表現例 **入院生活**

□面会時間と食事のスケジュールを教えてください。
Would you tell me the visiting hours and the schedule of meals?

□英語を話せる看護師さんはいますか。
Is there an English speaking nurse on the staff?

□担当医の診察はいつですか。
When will my doctor come to see me?

□偏頭痛がひどいので検査を休ませてください。
I'd like to skip the tests because I have a bad migraine now.

□外泊してもいいかを先生に聞いていただけますか。
Would you please ask my doctor if I could stay out overnight?

□お薬について説明していただけますか。
Will you please explain about my medication?

□1日中ベッドで寝ていなければなりませんか。
Do I have to stay in bed all day?

□部屋でなくカフェテリアで食事をしていいですか。
Can I eat in Cafeteria instead of in my room?

□5階の大きい部屋に移りたいのですが。
I'd like to be transferred to a bigger room on the fifth floor.

□ナースステーションの近くの部屋に移りたいのです。
I'd like to move to a room near the nurses' station.

③ 退院：Discharge

①6月15日に退院できます。
You can leave the hospital on June 15.

②術後の診察に必ず来てくださいね。
Be sure to keep your follow-up appointment.

③退院おめでとうございます。
Congratulations on getting out of the hospital.

④リハビリテーション施設にご紹介しておきました。
We have referred you to the rehabilitation facilities.

⑤食事を作ってくれる方がいますか。
Is there anyone who can prepare meals for you?

患者さんからの表現例　退院

□いつ退院できるか教えてください。
Please let me know when I can go home.

□家に帰れるようにどなたか手配してくれませんか。
Can someone help me with arrangements for going home?

④ Operation：手術

(a) Pre-Operation：手術前

①今までに手術をされたことはありますか。
Have you ever had any operations before?

②手術前にいくつか検査を受けていただきます。
You will have several examinations before the operation.

③主治医から手術の説明があります。
The doctor in charge will explain the operation to you.

④この同意書をよく読まれたうえでここにサインしてください。
Please read the consent form carefully, and sign here.

⑤手術は明日の朝10時からです。
The operation is scheduled for ten o'clock tomorrow morning.

⑥明日の朝の9時半に手術控え室(所)にお送りします。
We will take you to the pre-operation room (area) at nine thirty tomorrow morning.

⑦散髪をしておいてください。
Please have your hair cut.

⑧手術の前は食べたり飲んだりしてはいけません。
You cannot eat or drink before the operation.

⑨夕食後下剤を飲んでください。
Please take the laxatives after dinner.

⑩今晩お風呂に入ってください。
Please take a bath tonight.

⑪手術の前にシャワーを浴びるかお風呂に入っていただきます。
You have to take a shower or bath before the operation.

⑫全身（局所）麻酔を受けていただきます。
You will receive general (local) anesthesia.

⑬この手術ガウンを着てください。
Please wear this hospital gown.

⑭コンタクトレンズ（入れ歯，補聴器）をはずしてください。
Please take out your contact lenses (dentures; hearing aid).

⑮手術前にお腹の毛を剃ります。
We will shave your abdomen before the operation.

⑯このマスクをつけてください。
Please wear this mask.

患者さんからの表現例 **手術前**

□ 手術はいつになりますか。
When will my operation be scheduled?

□ 手術のためにいくつ検査を受けるのですか。
How many tests will I have before the operation?

□ 手術の前に食べていいのですか。
Can I eat before the operation?

□ とても緊張しています。
I am very nervous.

□ 手術を延期できますか。
Can you put off the operation?

□ 手術の後いつこの部屋に帰ってこれますか。
When will I come back to my room after the operation?

□ 手術中は目がさめているのですか。
Will I be awake during the operation?

□ 手術前に神父さんに会えますか。
Can I see the priest before my operation?

□ 術後痛みますか。
Will I be in pain after the surgery?

□ 術後どのぐらいで歩けるようになりますか。
When will I be able to walk after the operation?

□ 術後はしびんを使わなければならないのでしょうか。
Should I use the bedpan to pass water after the operation?

□ 術後リハビリが必要でしょうか。
Will I need rehabilitation after the operation (surgery)?

(b) Post-Operation：手術後

① 今あなたは回復室にいます。
You are in the recovery room now.

② 手術はうまく行きました。
The operation went well.

③ 1時間ほどしたら病室に戻れます。
You can return to your room in about an hour.

④ ガスが出たら教えてください。
Please let us know if you pass gas.

⑤ 数日間は流動食です。
You will be on a liquid diet for several days.

⑥ 水分と栄養のために点滴をします。
We will give you an intravenous drip for water and nutrients.

 患者さんからの表現例 **手術後**

□ 手術はうまくいきましたか。
Did the operation go well?

□ 手術はどうでしたか。
How did the surgery go?

□ どのような痛み止めをもらえますか。
What kind of painkiller will I get?

⑤ Daily Routine：日常生活

(a) Self-Introduction：自己紹介

①担当看護師の山田ルミです。
I am Rumi Yamada, your primary nurse.

②担当の医師は山本医師です。
Your doctor on this unit is Dr. Yamamoto.

③入ってもいいですか。
May I come in?

④すぐ戻ってきます。
I'll come back soon.

⑤また後ほど。
See you later.

⑥もう一度言っていただけますか。
Pardon〔me〕?

⑦もっとゆっくり話していただけますか。
Please speak more slowly.

⑧何か質問はありませんか。
Do you have any questions?

(b) Orientation：病棟案内

①この部屋は個室です。
This room is a private room.

②差額ベッド代をお支払いいただければ個室に移れます。
You can move to a private room, if you pay an additional charge.

③同じお部屋の方をご紹介します。
Let me introduce your roommates〔to you〕.

④ナースコールのテストをしましょう。
Let us try out the call button.

⑤看護師を呼ぶにはこのボタンをこのように押してください。
Push this button, like this, to call the nurse.

⑥この病棟をご案内しましょう。
Let me show you around this ward.

⑦ここへは入らないでください。
Please do not enter here.

⑧この表示は避難経路を示しています。
This sign shows the emergency escape route.

⑨エレベーターで9階に行ってください。
Take the elevator to the 9th floor.

⑩こちらのエスカレーターをお使いください。
Please use this escalator.

⑪売店は地下1階です。
The store is in the first basement.

⑫食堂は3階です。
The cafeteria is on the third floor.

⑬ナースステーションは階段の近くです。
The nurses' station is near the stairway.

⑭廊下をまっすぐ行って、右に曲がってください。
Go straight up the hall, and turn right.

⑮持ち物はロッカーに入れてください。
Please put your belongings in the locker.

⑯貴重品はお部屋に置かないでください。
Please do not leave valuables in the room.

⑰看護師は、午後4時, 12時, 午前8時の8時間ごとに交替します。
The nurses change shifts at 4:00 p.m., 12:00 p.m., and 8:00 a.m. We are on 8-hour shifts.

⑱電気器具は使用する前に許可を得てください。
Please request permission before using electrical appliances.

⑲コインランドリーがご利用いただけます。
We have a coin-operated laundry.

⑳院外へ出られるときにはお知らせください。
Please let us know if you will leave the hospital.

㉑月曜から金曜までの面会時間は午後2時から8時までです。
Visiting hours are from 2:00 p.m. to 8:00 p.m. on weekdays.

㉒あちらの公衆電話が使えます。
You can use the pay phone over there.

㉓公衆電話はテレフォンカードが使えます。
You can use the pay phone with a telephone card.

㉔病室で携帯電話を使ってはいけません。
You cannot use cell phones in the room.

㉕この案内書(パンフレット, 冊子)を読んでください。
Please read this guide (pamphlet; leaflet).

患者さんからの表現例　病棟案内

☐ナースコールはどのように使えばいいのですか。
How should I use the call button?

☐貴重品はどこにしまえばいいですか。
Where should I keep my valuables?

☐小銭で公衆電話がかけられますか。
Can I use the pay phone with coins?

☐外からの電話に出られますか。
Can I receive phone calls from outside?

☐病院からEメールを送ることができますか。
Can I send e-mail from this hospital?

☐個室料金はおいくらですか。
How much is the additional fee for a private room?

Hospital Personnel

医療従事者

Words and Terms 基本用語

① Administrators：管理職

1. hospital director — 院長
2. vice director — 副院長
3. director of nursing department — 看護部長
5. chief administrator — 事務長

② Nursing Department：看護部

8. supervisor — 管理師長
9. head nurse【米】; Sister【英】 — 病棟師長
10. clinical nurse specialist [CNS] — 専門看護師
12. registered nurse [RN] — 正看護師
13. charge nurse — 主任看護師
14. primary nurse — プライマリーナース
15. nurse practitiner [NP] — 特定看護師(一定レベルの診断や治療が許されている看護師)【米】
17. surgical nurse; scrub nurse — 手術専門看護師
19. night nurse — 夜間勤務の看護師
20. licensed practical nurse [LPN] — 准看護師

1	☐ nurse's aid; nursing assistant	看護助手
3	☐ **student nurse**	**看護実習生**
4	☐ orderly	看護補助員
5	☐ **midwife**	**助産師**
6	☐ visiting nurse	訪問看護師

③ Physician and Staff：医師，スタッフ

9	☐ **physician; doctor**	**医師**
10	☐ physician (doctor) in charge	主治医
12	☐ **general practitioner [GP]; family doctor; primary physician**	**一般開業医，家庭医**
15	☐ resident	研修医
16	☐ **pharmacist**	**薬剤師**
17	☐ medical social worker	医療ソーシャルワーカー
18	☐ **lab technician**	**臨床検査技師**
19	☐ **X-ray technician**	**X線技師**
20	☐ MRI technician	MRI技師
21	☐ PET technician	PET技師
22	☐ dietitian; nutritionist	栄養士
23	☐ **physical therapist [PT]**	**理学療法士**
24	☐ **occupational therapist [OT]**	**作業療法士**
26	☐ speech therapist	言語療法士
27	☐ clinical psychologist	臨床心理士
28	☐ music therapist	音楽療法士
29	☐ orthoptist	視能訓練士
30	☐ dental hygienist	歯科衛生士

医療従事者

1. ☐ dental technician 歯科技工士
2. ☐ clerk 事務職員
3. ☐ **receptionist** **受付係**
4. ☐ **cashier** **会計係**
5. ☐ volunteer ボランティア
6. ☐ **emergency medical technician [EMT]** **救急医療隊員**
8. ☐ paramedic 救急医療士, 医療補助員

④ Areas of Specialty and Specialists：専門と専門医

11. ☐ family medicine 家庭医学
12. ☐ internal medicine 内科
13. ☐ **internist** **内科医**
14. ☐ cardiology 循環器科
15. ☐ **cardiologist** **循環器専門医**
16. ☐ gastroenterology 消化器科
17. ☐ gastroenterologist 消化器専門医
18. ☐ pulmonology; respiratory medicine 呼吸器科
20. ☐ pulmonologist 呼吸器専門医
21. ☐ endocrinology 内分泌科
22. ☐ endocrinologist 内分泌専門医
23. ☐ surgery 外科
24. ☐ **surgeon** **外科医**
25. ☐ radiology 放射線科
26. ☐ radiologist 放射線科医
27. ☐ neurosurgery 脳神経外科
28. ☐ **neurosurgeon** **脳神経外科医**
29. ☐ orthopedics 整形外科
30. ☐ **orthopedist** **整形外科医**

2-02 Hospital Personnel

1. ☐ plastic surgery — 形成外科
2. ☐ plastic surgeon — 形成外科医
3. ☐ gynecology — 婦人科
4. ☐ **gynecologist** — **婦人科医**
5. ☐ obstetrics — 産科
6. ☐ **obstetrician** — **産科医**
7. ☐ pediatrics — 小児科
8. ☐ **pediatrician** — **小児科医**
9. ☐ psychiatry — 精神科
10. ☐ **psychiatrist** — **精神科医**
11. ☐ neurology — 神経科
12. ☐ neurologist — 神経科医
13. ☐ urology — 泌尿器科
14. ☐ **urologist** — **泌尿器科医**
15. ☐ otorhinolaryngology; ENT — 耳鼻咽喉科
16. (ear, nose, throat)
17. ☐ **otorhinolaryngologist;** — **耳鼻咽喉科医**
18. **ear, nose and throat**
19. **specialist**
20. ☐ ophthalmology — 眼科
21. ☐ **ophthalmologist; eye** — **眼科医**
22. **doctor**
23. ☐ dermatology — 皮膚科
24. ☐ **dermatologist** — **皮膚科医**
25. ☐ anesthesiology — 麻酔科
26. ☐ **anesthesiologist** — **麻酔科医**
27. ☐ dentistry — 歯科
28. ☐ **dentist** — **歯科医**
29. ☐ orthodontics — 矯正歯科
30. ☐ orthodontist — 矯正歯科医

Expressions 表現

① Reception：受付

①当院は初めてですか。
Is this your first visit to this hospital?

②ご予約はされていますか。
Do you have an appointment?

③呼ばれるまでの待ち時間にこの用紙に記入してください。
Please fill in this form while you are waiting to be called.

④診察券(保険証, 紹介状)はお持ちですか。
Do you have a hospital card (medical insurance card; letter of reference)?

⑤保険証を見せてください。
May I see your medical insurance card?

⑥すみませんが当院では外国の保険は扱えません。
I'm sorry we can't accept foreign insurance at our hospital.

⑦どちらの診療科を受診なさりたいですか。
Which department are you looking for?

⑧外科に行って診療券を窓口の箱にお入れください。
Please go to the surgical department and put your hospital card in the box at the counter.

⑨外来は午前中のみです。
The clinic is only open for outpatients in the morning.

⑩入院手続きについては病院事務でお聞きください。
Please ask about the procedure for admission at the hospital business office.

⑪医療ソーシャルワーカーかボランティアがお手伝いします。
The medical social worker or volunteer will help.

② Registration and Personal Profile：登録，個人情報

①最初に登録が必要です。
You'll need to register first.

②少しお伺いいたします。
Can you tell me a little about yourself.

③独身ですか，結婚していますか，別居ですか，離婚しましたか，それとも死別ですか。
Are you single, married, separated, divorced or widowed?

④ご職業は何でしょうか。
What is your occupation?

⑤近親者はどなたですか。
Who is your nearest relative?

⑥宗教は何でしょうか。
What is your religion?

⑦あなたの名前，年齢，生年月日，国籍を書いてください。
Please write your name, age, birth date, and nationality.

⑧あなたの現住所（本国の住所）と電話番号（勤務先の電話番号）を書いてください。
Please write your present (home) address and phone number (business phone number).

⑨緊急の連絡先はどなたですか。
Who is the person to be contacted in an emergency?

⑩その方の名前と関係を教えてください。
Can you tell me his (her) name and the relationship?

⑪日本語はいくらか話せますか。
Do you speak some Japanese?

⑫母国語は何ですか。
What's your native language?

医療従事者

③ Hospital Guide：院内案内

①当院の案内用地図です。
This is the guide map for this hospital.

②外科はお手洗いの隣です。
The surgery department is next to the restroom.

③院内レストランは地下です。
The hospital restaurant is in the basement.

④非常口はこの廊下の突き当たりです。
The emergency exit is at the end of this hall.

⑤内科は小児科と整形外科の間にあります。
Internal medicine is between pediatrics and orthopedics.

⑥皮膚科は3階ですので、そちらのエレベーターをお使いください。
Dermatology is on the third floor, so use that elevator over there.

⑦この階の薬局に行ってください。
Please go to the pharmacy on this floor.

⑧放射線室までご案内しましょう。
Let me take you to the radiology room.

④ Health Insurance and Payment：健康保険，支払い

①保険証をもっていますか。お見せください。
Do you have an insurance card? Please show it to me.

②保険がないとすべて自費支払いとなります。
If you do not have insurance, you'll have to pay all your medical charges.

③病院の費用は現金でのお支払いですか，それともカードですか。
How will you pay hospital charges, cash or credit card?

④支払いは会計でお願いします。
Please pay the hospital bill at the cashier.

⑤自動支払い機を使うこともできますよ。
You can use the automated payment machine.

⑥もし何か疑問があったら，受付でおたずねください。
If you have any questions, ask at the reception.

⑦次回に必ず診察券と保険証をご持参ください。
Please be sure to bring your hospital card and medical insurance card next time you come.

⑤ Appointment：予約

①今月は予約が一杯です。来月はいかがですか。
I am afraid I'm fully booked this month. How about next month?

②次回の予約をしてください。
Please make an appointment for the next time.

③受付で入院の予約をしてください。
Please make an appointment for hospitalization here at the admission office.

⑥ Medical Interview：問診，診察

(a) Basic expressions：基本表現

①今日の体調はいかがですか。
How do you feel today?

②どうなさいましたか。
What seems to be the problem?

③どこですか。
Where is it?

④いつ始まったのですか。
When did it start?

⑤それについて教えていただけますか。
Can you describe it for me?

⑥最近海外旅行に行きましたか。
Have you recently traveled anywhere out of Japan?

⑦いつ，どんな国へ旅行しましたか。
When and which countries did you go?

⑧どのように起こりますか。突然ですか，それとも徐々にですか。
How does it occur, suddenly or gradually?

⑨どのくらい続いていますか。
How long have you had it?

⑩起こる頻度はどのくらいですか。
How often does it occur?

⑪軽快傾向ですか，悪化傾向ですか，それとも変わりなしですか。
Is it getting better, getting worse, or the same?

⑫以前にもこの種の症状を経験したことはありましたか。
Have you had this kind of symptom before?

⑬思い当たる誘因はありましたか。
What do you think was causing it?

⑭他に思い当たる徴候や症状は何かありますか。
Have you noticed any other signs or symptoms?

⑮この前診察してから具合はいかがですか。
How have you been since I saw you last?

(b) Expressions at each department：各科での表現

①熱(頭痛, 鼻水, 喉頭炎, 発汗)がありますか。
Do you have a fever (a headache; a runny nose; a sore throat; sweating)?

②息切れあるいは胸の痛みはありますか。
Do you have shortness of breath, or chest pain?

③腹痛, 嘔吐, あるいは下痢がありますか。
Do you have abdominal pain, vomiting, or diarrhea?

④眼に緑内障のような問題がありましたか。
Have you ever had problems with your eyes such as glaucoma?

⑤最近食欲に変化がありましたか。
Have you had a change in your appetite recently?

⑥あなたの不安(体重減少, 体重増加)の原因は何だと思いますか。
What do you think is causing your anxiety (weight loss; weight gain)?

⑦目まいの発作はよくありますか。
Do you often have attacks of dizziness?

⑧家族に肝臓炎(結腸がん)になった人はいますか。
Has anyone in your immediate family had hepatitis (colon cancer)?

⑨排尿が困難ですか。
Do you have difficulty urinating?

(c) Expressions after the interview：診察後の表現

① あなたのケアプランを話しましょう。
Let me talk to you about our care plan.

② 脳(循環器)専門医に診てもらう必要がありますね。
You need to see a brain (heart) specialist.

③ よろこんで紹介状を書きますよ。
I'm happy to write a referral letter.

④ 他の病棟(病院)に紹介しましょう。
Let me refer you to another unit (hospital).

⑤ リハビリ医がその手術に関してもっと詳細に説明してくれるでしょう。
The rehabilitation doctor will explain about the surgery in more detail.

⑥ 看護師から輸血に関するパンフレット(同意書)をお渡しします。
The nurse will give you the brochure (consent form) about blood transfusion.

⑦ 退院後,訪問看護婦がケアプランを作成します。
After discharge, the visiting nurse will make your care plan.

⑧ もしアレルギーがあるなら,栄養士(栄養学者)がそれに合わせた特別食を作ります。
If you have any allergies, the dietitians (nutritionists) will make a special diet for you.

Medications

薬剤

Words and Terms　基本用語

① General Terms：一般用語

- ☐ *quaque die*[*q.d.*]; once a day; every day　　1日1回, 毎日
- ☐ *bis in die*[*b.i.d.*]; twice a day　　1日2回
- ☐ *ter in die*[*t.i.d.*]; three times a day　　1日3回
- ☐ *quarter in die*[*q.d.s.*]; four times a day　　1日4回
- ☐ *quaque; quisque*; every [*q, Q*]　　〜ごと
- ☐ *omni hora*[*Oh*]; every hour　　1時間ごと
- ☐ **every other day**[*QOD*]　　隔日
- ☐ every week[*QW*]　　毎週
- ☐ *pro re nata*[*p.r.n.*]; **as necessary**　　必要に応じて
- ☐ *ante cibum; ante cibos*[*a.c.*]; **before meals**　　食前
- ☐ *post cibum; post cibos*[*p.c.*]; **after meals**　　食後
- ☐ *inter cibos*[*i.c.*]　　食間

薬剤

#		
1	☐ **during a meal; with meals**	食事中
3	☐ when hungry	空腹時
4	☐ *hora somni* [*h.s.*]; at bedtime	就眠時
6	☐ *semissem* [*ss*]; a half	半分
7	☐ spoonful	スプーン1杯
8	☐ **dose; dosage [dos.]**	**投薬量**
9	☐ maximum dose	極量
10	☐ lethal dose [LD]	致死量
11	☐ effective dose [ED]	有効量
12	☐ over dose [OD]	過量
13	☐ *separandum*	劇薬
14	☐ **side effect**	**副作用**
15	☐ Chinese herbal medicine	漢方薬
16	☐ household medicine	家庭常備薬
17	☐ **over-the-counter medicine [OTC]**	**市販薬**
19	☐ magic bullet	特効薬
20	☐ analeptic	気付け薬
21	☐ placebo	偽薬(ぎやく), プラセボ
22	☐ nutritional supplement	栄養剤
23	☐ preventive medicine	予防薬
24	☐ lifesaving drug	救急薬
25	☐ **vaccine**	**ワクチン**
26	☐ vitamin drops	ビタミン剤
27	☐ wafer	オブラート
28	☐ **prescription [Rx]**	**処方箋**
29	☐ **pharmacy**	**薬局**
30	☐ allergy	アレルギー

② Route of Administration：形態，用法

(a) oral：経口

☐ powdered medicine	粉薬・散剤
☐ **tablet[Tab]**	**錠剤**
☐ **granule**	**顆粒剤**
☐ capsule[Cap]	カプセル
☐ **pill**	**丸薬**
☐ liquid medicine	水薬
☐ lozenge	トローチ剤
☐ sublingual medication	舌下製剤
☐ **syrup[syr]**	**シロップ剤**

(b) external：外用

☐ **ointment[oit]**	**軟膏**
☐ cream	クリーム剤
☐ plaster	膏薬
☐ powder	パウダー剤
☐ spray	スプレー剤
☐ suppository[supp]	坐薬
☐ **inhalent**	**吸入薬**
☐ **eye-drops**	**点眼薬**
☐ nose drops	点鼻薬
☐ solution[sol]	溶液
☐ water[aq.]	水
☐ saline; normal saline[NS]	生理食塩液

③ Types of Medications：薬の種類

cold medicine	風邪薬
cough medicine	**咳止め薬**
cough syrup	咳止めシロップ
gargle; mouthwash	うがい薬
anti-flu medicine	インフルエンザ治療薬
expectorant	去痰薬
antibiotic	**抗生物質**
bronchodilator	気管支拡張薬
bronchoconstrictor	気管支収縮薬
antiasthmatic	喘息治療薬
painkiller	**鎮痛剤**
antipyretic	解熱薬
antiphlogistic	消炎薬
antimycotic agent	抗真菌薬
diuretic	利尿薬
antidiuretic	抗利尿薬
digestive medicine	**胃腸薬**
antiflatulent	整腸剤
digestive	消化剤
antiacid	制酸剤
laxative	**緩下剤**
antidiarrhetic	下痢止め薬
emetic	吐薬（嘔吐を引き起こす薬）
antiemetic	制吐薬
hepatic stimulant	強肝薬
anthelmintic	駆虫薬（腸内から寄生虫を駆除する薬）
antihypertensive	**抗高血圧薬**

2-03 Medications

1. ☐ cardiotonic agent — 強心剤
2. ☐ cholesterol-lowering agent — コレステロール降下薬
3. ☐ anticoagulant — 抗血液凝固薬
4. ☐ blood coagulation inhibitor — 血液凝固阻止薬
5. ☐ vasodilator — 血管拡張薬
6. ☐ vasoconstrictor — 血管収縮薬
7. ☐ antianemic agent — 抗貧血薬
8. ☐ **anesthetic** — **麻酔薬**
9. ☐ carcinostatic; cyto-toxic — 抗がん剤
10. ☐ immunosuppressant — 免疫抑制剤
11. ☐ antidote — 解毒剤
12. ☐ hematinic — 造血薬
13. ☐ muscle relaxer — 筋肉弛緩薬
14. ☐ antipruritic — かゆみ止め
15. ☐ antiallergic agent — 抗アレルギー薬
16. ☐ **steroid** — **ステロイド**
17. ☐ **histaminergic drug** — **ヒスタミン薬**
18. ☐ antihistamines — 抗ヒスタミン薬
19. ☐ hormonal drug — ホルモン薬
20. ☐ melanin blocker — メラニン阻害薬
21. ☐ topical medicine — 局所薬
22. ☐ **rubbing alcohol** — **消毒用アルコール**
23. ☐ antiseptic — 消毒剤, 防腐剤
24. ☐ iodine tincture — ヨードチンキ

Expressions 表現

①薬が3種類出ています。
You have three kinds of medicine.

②錠剤を2個ずつ,食後1日3回飲んでください。
Take two tablets three times a day, after each meal.

③毎食後30分以内に飲んでください。
Take this medicine within 30 minutes of eating each meal.

④この薬を朝食と一緒にお飲みください。
Take this pill with breakfast.

⑤1回1錠,痛いときに飲んでください。
Take one tablet at a time when you have a pain.

⑥この薬を1日2回2週間続けて服用してください。
Take this medicine twice a day for 2 weeks.

⑦痛み止めを持ってきました。
I brought you a pain killer.

⑧気分がよくなったらこの薬を飲むのをやめてもいいです。
You can stop taking this medicine, if you get better.

⑨お薬のアレルギーはありますか。
Do you have any drug allergies?

⑩この軟膏を塗ってください。
Please apply this ointment.

⑪これは座薬です。肛門から挿入します。
This is a suppository. It is to be inserted into the anus.

⑫かゆみが出たら中止してください。
Please stop taking (using) this medicine if you feel itchy.

⑬目薬をさしてください。
Please use〔these〕eye drops.

患者さんからの表現例 投薬

□ 私はアスピリンアレルギーです。
I'm allergic to aspirin.

□ 薬は1日何回飲めばいいのですか。
How many times a day should I take this medicine?

□ これは何の薬ですか。
What's this medicine for?

□ この薬はまったく効きません。
This medicine doesn't work at all.

□ この薬を飲むと頭痛がしますが、飲み続けなくてはいけないですか。
I have a headache after taking this medicine. Should I continue taking it?

□ このお薬にはどのような副作用がありますか。
What side effects does this medicine have?

□ 薬を飲んだあと発疹がでました。
I got rashes after taking this medicine.

□ お薬を変えてもらえませんか。
Will you change my medicine?

2-04 Daily Activities of Patients

患者さんの日常生活

Words and Terms 基本用語

① Daily Actions：日々の行為

1. ☐ blink — まばたきする
2. ☐ blow one's nose — 鼻をかむ
3. ☐ burp — げっぷをする
4. ☐ **chew** — **噛む**
5. ☐ dream — 夢をみる
6. ☐ drool — よだれをたらす
7. ☐ doze off; take a nap — 居眠りをする
8. ☐ **hiccup** — しゃっくりをする
9. ☐ **pass gas** — おならをならす
10. ☐ stretch — 伸びる
11. ☐ **swallow** — **飲み込む**
12. ☐ **sweat** — **汗をかく**
13. ☐ talk in one's sleep — 寝言をいう
14. ☐ yawn — あくびをする

② Eating：食事

17. ☐ breakfast/lunch/supper — 朝食／昼食／夕食
18. ☐ mealtime — 食事時間
19. ☐ **general diet** — **普通食**
20. ☐ special diet — 特別食
21. ☐ **gruel** — **粥**
22. ☐ rice — 米

1	bread	パン
2	liquid diet	流動食
3	**tube feeding**	**経管栄養**
4	soft diet	軟らかい食事, 軽食
5	**solid diet**	**固形食**
6	therapeutic diet	治療食
7	post operative diet	術後食
8	**cardiac diet**	**心臓病食**
9	**renal disease diet**	**腎臓病食**
10	**diabetic diet**	**糖尿病食**
11	low-salt diet	減塩食
12	**salt-free diet**	**無塩食**
13	sugar-free diet	無糖食
14	high-protein diet	高タンパク食
15	liquids; fluids	水分
16	**vegetarian**	**菜食主義者**
17	seasoning	味付け, 調味料
18	snack between meals	間食
19	dish	皿
20	bowl	椀
21	chopsticks	はし
22	tooth pick	つまようじ
23	tray	トレイ
24	**cart; wagon**	**ワゴン**
25	preparation for eating	摂食準備
26	setting for meal	食事のセッティング
27	help with eating	食事介助
28	**hydration**	**水分補給**

③ Grooming and Cleanliness：身づくろい

- **brushing; tooth brushing**　　**歯磨き**
- toothbrush　　歯ブラシ
- toothpaste　　練り歯磨き剤
- face washing　　洗顔
- wash-basin　　洗面器
- cleansing cream　　洗顔クリーム
- **skin lotion**　　**化粧水**
- makeup　　化粧
- **soap**　　**石鹸**
- towel　　タオル
- hair brush　　ヘアブラシ
- hair comb　　くし
- styling　　整髪
- **shaving**　　**ひげを剃ること**
- shaver　　〔電気〕かみそり
- razor　　かみそり
- shaving foam　　ひげそりクリーム
- toiletries　　洗面用具
- **haircut**　　**散髪**
- nailclipper　　爪切り
- **bed bath[BB]; sponge-bath**　　**清拭**（せいしき：ベッドの上で体を洗うこと）
- bath　　入浴
- hand bath　　手浴
- foot bath [FB]　　足浴
- bath towel　　バスタオル
- **shampoo**　　**洗髪**
- shower cap　　シャワーキャップ

1. **faucet** — 蛇口
2. bathtub — 浴槽
3. dryer — ドライヤー
4. **detergent** — **洗剤**
5. laundry — 洗濯物
6. laundry bag — 洗濯物袋
7. **help with bath** — **入浴介助**
8. help with shower — シャワー浴介助

④ Excretion：排泄

11. **urination** — 排尿
12. **urine** — **尿**
13. **bowel movement(s)** — **排便**
14. **stool** — **大便**
15. toilet — トイレ
16. **occupied** — 〔トイレなどが〕使用中
17. emergency buzzer — 非常用ベル
18. **bedpan** — 〔病人用〕便器
19. commode — カモード（洋式の室内用トイレ）
20. toilet paper — トイレットペーパー
21. tissue — ティッシュペーパー
22. **help using the toilet (commode; bedpan)** — **排泄介助**

⑤ Sleep：睡眠

- **wake-up time** — 起床時間
- **lights-out time** — 消灯時間
- pajamas — パジャマ
- **blanket** — 毛布
- sheet — シーツ
- **pillow** — 枕
- bedclothes — 寝具
- flashlight — 懐中電灯
- **nap** — 昼寝
- preparation for sleeping — 就寝の準備
- help with falling sleep — 入眠介助
- adjustment of sleep pattern — 睡眠パターンの調整

⑥ Personal Belongings：身周り品

- **false teeth; dentures** — 入れ歯, 義歯
- (a pair of eye) glasses — メガネ
- contact lenses — コンタクトレンズ
- wig — かつら
- (a pair of) slippers — スリッパ
- clothing — 衣類
- **underwear** — 下着
- brassiere [bra] — ブラジャー
- apron — エプロン
- button — ボタン
- accessory — アクセサリー
- **valuables** — 貴重品
- metalic items — 金属製の物

#		
1	☐ **cell phone**	携帯電話
2	☐ **garbage bag**	ゴミ袋
3	☐ trash box	ゴミ箱
4	☐ dustcloth	雑巾
5	☐ electrical appliance	電気器具

⑦ Others：その他

#		
8	☐ **visiting hours**	面会時間
9	☐ **visitor**	見舞い人
10	☐ **stay out overnight**	外泊する
11	☐ go out	外出する
12	☐ dressing	更衣
13	☐ sun bathe	日光浴
14	☐ exercise	運動
15	☐ **consent form**	同意書
16	☐ **health insurance card**	健康保険証
17	☐ **(hospital) ID card**	身分証明書(診察券)

---

column **ことわざ２**

☐ 健全な精神は健全な身体に宿る
　Sound mind in a sound body.
☐ 人生とはただ生きることでなく楽しむことである
　Life consists not in breathing but in enjoying life.
☐ 心配は身の毒
　Care killed a cat. / Worry often causes illness.
☐ 生命あるかぎり希望あり
　While there is life there is hope.
☐ 風邪は万病のもと
　Everything starts with a cold.

Expressions 表現

① Eating:食事

①毎日,朝食は8時,昼食は12時,夕食は6時です。
Breakfast is served at 8, lunch at noon, and supper at 6 every day.

②トレイはご自分でワゴンにお返しください。
Please return the tray to the cart.

③明日から普通食です。
You will have a general diet from tomorrow on.

④病院食以外は食べないでください。
Please do not eat anything except for hospital meals.

⑤どのぐらい食べたか教えてください。
Let us know how much you ate.

⑥昼食はおいしかったですか。
Did you enjoy your lunch?

⑦アルコール類は飲まないでください。
You cannot drink alcohol.

⑧宗教によって食べられないものがあったらお知らせください。
If there are any foods you cannot eat for religious reasons, please tell us (me) now.

⑨入院中,毎日糖尿病食(心臓病食)です。
You will have the diabetic diet (cardiac diet) every day during your hospitalization.

患者さんからの表現例 **食事**

☐ 牡蠣アレルギーがあります。
I am allergic to oysters.

☐ 宗教上お肉が食べられません。
I cannot eat meat for religious reasons.

☐ 食後食器はどうすればいいですか。
What should I do with my dishes after meals?

☐ 病院食以外何を食べてもいいですか。
Can I eat anything in addition to hospital meals?

② Excretion:排泄

① ここがトイレです。
This is the toilet (bathroom).

② 洗濯場は別になっています。
The sink for washing is in a separate area.

③ トイレで気分が悪くなったらこの緊急連絡ブザーを押してください。
Please push the emergency button if you feel sick while in the rest room.

④ トイレに行けないときは呼んでください。お連れします。
Please call us if you cannot get to the toilet. We will help you.

⑤ 夜トイレに行けないときはカモードをお使いください。
If you cannot get to the toilet at night, you can use this commode.

⑥ カモードというのは洋式の室内用トイレです。
A commode chair is a kind of chair with a chamberpot.

⑦術後は便器を使っていただきます。
You will have to use a bedpan after the operation.

 患者さんからの表現例　排泄

□トイレに1人で行っていいですか。
Can I go to the toilet alone?

□便器を使用した後どうすればいいですか。
What should I do after using the bedpan?

□何度もトイレに行きたくなり目が覚めます。
I wake up to go to the toilet many times.

□便が緩いです。
I have loose bowels.

□尿がいくらか漏れます。
Sometimes I leak some urine.

③ Bathing 入浴

①ここがお風呂です。
This is the bath.

②男性は火,木,土曜日に入浴できます。
Men can bathe on Tuesdays, Thursdays and Saturdays.

③入浴は午前9時〜午後9時までいつでもできます。
You can take a bath anytime from 9:00 a.m. to 9:00 p.m.

④あまり長時間お風呂(シャワー)に入らないでください。
Don't take too much time in the bath (shower).

⑤熱があるときはお風呂やシャワーに入れません。
You can't take a bath or shower when you have a fever.

⑥タオルとシャンプーはお持ちですか。
Do you have a bath towel and shampoo?

⑦ここを右に回してください。お湯が出ます。
Turn this clockwise. Hot water will come out.

⑧髪を洗いましょうか。
Shall I shampoo your hair?

患者さんからの表現例 入浴

□お風呂に入っていいですか。
Can I take a bath?

□お風呂に入る手伝いをしてもらえますか。
Will you help me to take a bath?

□足を洗ってもらえますか。
Will you help me to wash my feet?

□髪を乾かしてもらえますか。
Will you dry my hair?

④ Sleep：睡眠

①消灯時間は午後10時です。
Lights-out is 10:00 p.m.

②寝る時間ですよ。
It's time to sleep.

③よく眠ってください。
Please sleep well.

④電気を消してください。
Please turn off the light.

⑤昨晩はよく眠れましたか。
Did you sleep well last night?

⑥気分を楽にするために何かして差し上げましょうか。
What can I do to make you more comfortable?

⑦痛みが取れればよく眠れるようになります。
You should sleep better when the pain is gone.

⑧痛み止めが必要ですか。
Do you think you need some pain medication now?

⑨真夜中にしばしば目が覚めるようなら教えてください。
Please let us know if you wake up often during the night.

⑩消灯時刻以降は眠るように努力してみてください。
After lights-out, please try to sleep.

患者さんからの表現例　睡眠

□眠れません。ここは騒がしすぎます。
　I can't get to sleep. It's too noisy here.

□眠れないときは睡眠薬を飲んでいいですか。
　Can I take sleeping pills when I can't sleep?

□痛みがひどくて眠れません。
　It hurts so much that I can't sleep.

□夜何度も目が覚めます。
　I wake up many times during the night.

□息が詰まるような感じがして目が覚めます。
　I wake up feeling I can't breathe.

PART 3
解剖・徴候・疾患の基本用語と表現

3-01

External Body Parts

身体の外部

Words and Terms 基本用語

1. **head** — 頭, 頭部
2. hair — 頭髪
3. **face** — 顔
4. forehead — 額
5. temple — こめかみ
6. **eye** — 目
7. eyebrow — 眉
8. eyelid — 瞼(まぶた)
9. upper lid / lower lid — 上まぶた／下まぶた
10. eyelash — 睫毛(まつげ)
11. **cheek** — ほお
12. **nose** — 鼻
13. nostril — 鼻孔
14. **ear / (ear) lobe** — 耳／耳たぶ
15. **mouth** — 口
16. lip — 唇
17. upper lip / lower lip — 上唇／下唇
18. **jaw** — 顎
19. **chin** — 下顎
20. **neck** — 首
21. nape of neck — 襟首, 首筋
22. Adam's apple — のどぼとけ
23. **shoulder** — 肩

身体の外部

1	☐ **chest; rib cage; thorax**	胸
2	☐ **armpit**	わきの下
3	☐ armpit hair	わき毛
4	☐ nipple	乳首
5	☐ **breast**	**乳房**
6	☐ **back**	背中
7	☐ **abdomen[abd]; belly;**	腹
8	**tummy**	
9	☐ side	わき腹
10	☐ waist	ウエスト
11	☐ navel; belly button;	へそ
12	umbilicus	
13	☐ arm	腕
14	☐ upper arm	上腕
15	☐ **elbow**	肘
16	☐ forearm	前腕
17	☐ wrist	手首
18	☐ hand	手
19	☐ palm	手のひら
20	☐ back of the hand	手の甲
21	☐ knuckle	指関節
22	☐ **finger nail**	**指の爪**
23	☐ nail bed; lunula	半月
24	☐ **thumb**	**親指**
25	☐ **index finger**	人差し指
26	☐ middle finger	中指
27	☐ ring finger	薬指
28	☐ little finger; pinky	小指
29	☐ groin	脚の付け根, 股間, 鼠径部
30	☐ **buttocks**	**殿部**

1	☐ **genitals**	生殖器
2	☐ thigh	大腿部
3	☐ **leg**	脚
4	☐ **knee**	膝
5	☐ **shin**	すね
6	☐ **calf**	ふくらはぎ
7	☐ ankle	足首
8	☐ heel	かかと
9	☐ **foot**	足
10	☐ sole	足の裏
11	☐ top of the foot	足の甲
12	☐ toe	足指
13	☐ big toe / little toe	足の親指／小指
14	☐ toenail	足指の爪

Expressions 表現

①筋肉,関節,骨の具合が悪いですか。
Are you having troubles in any of your muscles, joints, or bones?

②首(背中)に悪いところはありますか。
Is there anything wrong with your neck (back)?

③今までにどこか骨折したことがありますか。
Have you ever broken any bones?

④膝(肘,手首)を曲げたり,伸ばしたりしてください。
Bend and stretch your knees (elbows; wrists).

⑤この手すりをしっかり握ってください。
Grip this rail tightly.

⑥足(腕)を上げてください。
Raise your legs. (arms).

患者さんからの表現例 主訴

☐ 2日前に転倒しました。
I had a fall two days ago.

☐ 寝違えました。
I have a crick in my neck from sleeping wrong.

☐ 足元がふらつきます。
I feel shaky on my feet.

☐ 足の甲に腫れがあるのに気付きました。
I have noticed some swelling on the top of my feet.

☐ まぶたの具合が悪く,眼を閉じることができないのです。
Something may be wrong with my eyelids.
I can't close my eyes.

Internal Body Parts

身体の内部

Words and Terms 基本用語

① Skeletal System：骨格系

1. **bone** — 骨
2. skull — 頭蓋
3. **cervical vertebra** — 頸椎
4. **spine** — 背骨, 脊椎
5. collar bone; clavicle — 鎖骨
6. **shoulder blade; scapula** — 肩甲骨
7. 【単】, **scapulae**【複】
8. breastbone; sternum — 胸骨
9. **rib** — 肋骨
10. thoracic vertebra — 胸椎
11. lumbar vertebra — 腰椎
12. humerus【単】, humeri【複】 — 上腕骨
13. ulna【単】, ulnae【複】 — 尺骨
14. radius【単】, radii【複】 — 橈骨（とうこつ）
15. carpus【単】, carpi【複】 — 手根骨
16. metacarpal — 中手骨
17. phalanx【単】, phalanges【複】 — 指節骨
18. **pelvis** — 骨盤
19. pelvic bone — 寛骨
20. sacrum【単】, sacra【複】 — 仙骨
21. coccyx【単】, coccyges【複】 — 尾骨
22. femur【単】, femora【複】 — 大腿骨

1	☐ **kneecap; patella**【単】,	膝蓋骨(しつがいこつ)
2	**patellae**【複】	
3	☐ fibula	腓骨(ひこつ)
4	☐ tibia【単】, tibiae【複】	脛骨(けいこつ)
5	☐ tarsus【単】, tarsi【複】	足根骨
6	☐ metatarsal	中足骨

② Muscular and Joint System：筋，関節系

- ☐ **muscle** — 筋肉
- ☐ **joint** — 関節
- ☐ tendon — 腱
- ☐ **Achilles' tendon** — アキレス腱
- ☐ ligament — 靭帯
- ☐ sphincter — 括約筋

③ Brain and Nervous System：脳，神経系

- ☐ **brain** — 脳
- ☐ brainstem — 脳幹
- ☐ **cerebrum** — 大脳
- ☐ **cerebellum** — 小脳
- ☐ spinal cord — 脊髄
- ☐ meninx【単】, meninges【複】 — 髄膜
- ☐ **nerve** — 神経
- ☐ **sympathetic nerve** — 交感神経
- ☐ **parasympathetic nerve** — 副交感神経
- ☐ **peripheral nerve** — 末梢神経
- ☐ trigeminal nerve — 三叉神経
- ☐ optic nerve — 視神経
- ☐ sciatic nerve — 坐骨神経

④ Respiratory System：呼吸器系

- **throat** 咽喉
- pharynx【単】, pharynges【複】 咽頭
- larynx【単】, larynges【複】 喉頭
- uvula 口蓋垂
- **tonsil** 扁桃腺
- epiglottis 喉頭蓋
- **vocal cords** 声帯
- **trachea**【単】, **tracheae**【複】 気管
- bronchus【単】, bronchi【複】 気管支
- **lung** 肺
- diaphragm 横隔膜

⑤ Circulatory System：循環器系

- **heart** 心臓
- **blood vessel** 血管
- capillary 毛細血管
- **valve** 弁
- left atrium [LA] 左心房
- left ventricle [LV] 左心室
- right atrium [RA] 右心房
- right ventricle [RV] 右心室
- apex cordis 心尖
- aorta【単】, aortae【複】 大動脈
- superior vena cava 上大静脈
- **coronary artery** 冠状動脈
- inferior vena cava 下大静脈

⑥ Digestive System：消化器系

- **tongue** 舌
- taste buds 味覚芽, 味蕾(みらい)
- **saliva** 唾液
- **esophagus** 食道
- **stomach** 胃
- gastric juice 胃液
- **liver** 肝臓
- gallbladder[GB] 胆のう
- **pancreas** 膵臓
- small intestine 小腸
- duodenum 十二指腸
- jejunum 空腸
- ileum 回腸
- **large intestine** 大腸
- ascending colon 上行結腸
- transverse colon 横行結腸
- descending colon 下行結腸
- sigmoid colon S状結腸
- rectum 直腸
- cecum【単】, ceca【複】 盲腸
- appendix 虫垂
- **anus** 肛門

⑦ Urinary and Reproductive Systems：腎・泌尿器, 生殖器系

- **kidney** 腎臓
- urethra 尿道
- ureter 尿管
- **urinary bladder** 膀胱

1. **womb; uterus** — 子宮
2. **vagina** — 腟
3. ovary — 卵巣
4. placenta — 胎盤
5. amniotic fluid — 羊水
6. testicle — 睾丸
7. **penis** — 陰茎
8. **prostate gland** — 前立腺

⑧ Ear, Nose, Throat and Eye：耳，鼻，咽喉，眼

(a) sight：視覚

12. **eyeball** — **眼球**
13. cornea — 角膜
14. sclera【単】, scleras; sclerae【複】 — 強膜
16. conjunctiva — 結膜
17. pupil — 瞳孔
18. iris — 虹彩
19. lens — 水晶体
20. vitreous body — 硝子体
21. **retina** — **網膜**
22. tear duct — 涙管

(b) hearing：聴覚

24. auricle — 耳介
25. antihelix — 対耳輪
26. concha of auricle — 耳甲介
27. external ear — 外耳
28. external acoustic meatus — 外耳道
29. **eardrum** — **鼓膜**
30. middle ear — 中耳

1	☐ internal ear	内耳
2	☐ auditory tube	耳管
3	**(c) smell：嗅覚**	
4	☐ **nasal cavity**	**鼻腔**
5	☐ nasal septum	鼻中隔

⑨ Skin：皮膚

8	☐ epidermis	表皮
9	☐ dermis	真皮
10	☐ subcutaneous tissue	皮下組織
11	☐ **sweat gland**	**汗腺**
12	☐ sebaceous gland	皮脂腺
13	☐ **pore**	毛穴
14	☐ hair root	毛根
15	☐ hair bulb	毛球

⑩ Dentistry：歯科

18	☐ **tooth【単】, teeth【複】**	**歯**
19	☐ **gums; gum tissue**	**歯茎**
20	☐ baby tooth / permanent tooth	乳歯／永久歯
22	☐ wisdom tooth	親知らず, 智歯
23	☐ canine tooth; eye tooth	犬歯
24	☐ incisor	切歯(せっし)
25	☐ molar	臼歯(きゅうし)
26	☐ **front tooth / back tooth**	前歯／奥歯

⑪ Endocrine System：内分泌系

- **pituitary gland; hypophysis**　下垂体
- pineal gland　松果腺
- **thyroid gland**　甲状腺
- parathyroid gland　副甲状腺
- adrenal gland　副腎
- **thymus gland**　胸腺

⑫ Blood and Immune System：血液, 免疫系

- **white blood cell; leukocyte**　白血球
- **red blood cell; erythrocyte**　赤血球
- plasma　血漿
- platelet　血小板
- lymph　リンパ
- **lymphocyte**　リンパ球
- lymph gland / lymph node　リンパ腺／リンパ節
- T-cell; T lymphocyte　T 細胞
- natural killer cell [NK cell]　ナチュラルキラー細胞
- induced pluripotent stem cell [iPS cell]　iPS 細胞（人工多能性幹細胞）
- bone marrow　骨髄
- **spleen**　脾臓

Expressions 表現

① Skeletal System：骨格系

①右肩が脱臼しています。
You have dislocated your right shoulder.

②腕にギプスをします。
We'll put your arm in a plaster cast.

③首(腰部)の牽引をしましょう。
We'll need to put your neck (lower back) in traction.

④おじいさまは骨粗しょう症の治療が必要です。
Your grandfather needs treatment for his osteoporosis.

② Muscular and Joint System：筋，関節系

①流水で関節をよく冷やしましたか。
Did you cool the joint well with running water?

②コルセット(サポーター)をしましょう。
You will need to wear a corset (supporter).

③しばらく重いものは持たないでください。
Don't try to lift anything heavy for a while.

④筋肉が硬直と弛緩を繰り返しますか。
Do your muscles contract and relax by turn?

③ Brain and Nervous System：脳，神経系

①意識を失ったことがありますか。
Have you lost consciousness?

②痙攣を起こしたことがありますか。
Have you had convulsions or spasms?

③彼女は同じ質問を何度も繰り返すことがありますか。
Does she repeat the same questions many times?

④彼女は最近よく迷子になったりしますか。
Has she been getting lost a lot lately?

⑤彼女はよく物忘れをしますか。
Is she forgetful?

④ Respiratory System：呼吸器系

①呼吸に問題がありましたか。
Have you had any trouble with breathing?

②どんな痰が出ますか。
What kind of phlegm do you cough up?

③煙草を吸いますか。1日どのくらいか教えてください。
Do you smoke? How often do you smoke a day?

④まだ扁桃腺は残っているのですね。
Do you still have your tonsils?

⑤風邪から気管支を起こしています。
Your cold has developed into bronchitis.

⑤ Circulatory System：循環器系

①心臓の鼓動が不規則なことがありましたか。
Have you noticed any irregularities with your heart beat?

②どのような感じですか，非常に激しいですか，それとも不規則な感じですか。
What does it feel like, particularly fast, or irregular?

③その症状は運動後に起きますか，それとも安静にしているときですか。
Do you have the symptom after exercise or while resting?

④高血圧，高脂血症，あるいは糖尿病などの問題はありますか。
Do you have any problems, such as high blood pressure, hyperlipidemia, or diabetes?

⑤ストレスを感じたときに動悸がありますか。
Does your heart pound when you are stressed?

⑥ご家族の中に心筋梗塞や狭心症の方はいますか。
Has anyone in your family had a heart attack or angina pectoris?

⑦お気の毒ですが，お母さまは心不全のようです。
I'm sorry but your mother seems to be experiencing heart failure.

患者さんからの表現例　循環器

□しばしば手や指が震えます。
I often have trembling or shaking of my hands and fingers.

⑥ **Digestive System**：消化器系

①胸やけ(胃痛)がよくありますか。
Do you often feel heartburn (stomachache)?

②空腹時に胃が痛みますか。
Do you have a stomachache when you are hungry?

③胃液検査をしてみましょう。
Let's take a sample of your gastric juice.

④消化性潰瘍のようですね。
You seem to have a peptic ulcer.

⑤何回吐きましたか。
How many times did you throw up?

⑥何回下痢をしましたか。
How many times did you have diarrhea?

⑦いつも消化不良(膨満感)で苦しいですか。
Do you always suffer from indigestion (bloated feeling)?

⑧腸で最も心配しているのはどんなことですか。
What worries you most about your bowels?

 患者さんからの表現例 **消化器**

□食後にはずっとよくなります。
After meals, I feel much better.

⑦ Urinary and Reproductive Systems：腎・泌尿器，生殖器系

①膀胱のあたりが痛みますか。
Do you have pain around your bladder?

②いつもより頻繁におしっこが出ますか。
Do you need to urinate more often than usual?

③尿漏れはありますか。
Do you ever suffer from an involuntary discharge of urine?

④尿道にカテーテルをつけましょう。
You'll need to use a urinary catheter.

⑤この症状は腎炎ですね。
This symptom is from kidney inflammation.

⑥尿に血が混じっていたことはありますか。
Have you noticed blood in your urine?

⑦便通は規則的にありますか。
Do you have regular bowel movements?

⑧便秘しがちですか。
Do you tend to have constipation?

⑨局部にかゆみがありますか。
Do you feel itchy around your genitals?

⑩月経はいつも不規則ですか。
Are your periods usually irregular?

⑪月経間に出血はありますか。
Do you ever bleed between your periods?

⑫黒味をおびた褐色のおりものがありますか。
Do you have dark brown vaginal discharge?

⑬避妊はしていますか。
Do you practice birth control?

⑭性交中に痛みや不快感がありますか。
Do you feel any pain or discomfort during intercourse?

⑮閉経後, イライラや不安のような気分のむらがありますか。
Do you have mood swings such as irritability or nervousness after your menopause?

> ⑧ **Ear, Nose, Throat and Eye**：耳, 鼻, 咽喉, 眼

①私のことががはっきり見えますか。
Can you see me clearly?

②目がかすみますか。
Do you have blurred vision?

③指は何本見えますか。
How many fingers do you see?

④目やにに関するお悩みがありますか。
Have you been troubled by eye discharge?

⑤光が眩しいですか。
Are your eyes sensitive to light?

⑥視力検査をしましょう。
We will give you a vision test.

⑦1日何時間くらいコンタクトレンズを使用していますか。
How long do you wear your contact lenses each day?

⑧あまり長時間コンタクトレンズを使用し続けないでください。
Don't leave your contact lenses in for too long.

⑨網膜剥離がひどいですね。
Your retinal detachment is severe.

⑩舌を出してください。
Stick out your tongue, please.

⑪ナインナインと繰り返し言ってください。【欧米での従来からの診察方法】
Say " 99" over and over.

⑫鼻汁に血が見つかりました。
I found blood in my nasal discharge.

⑬急性篇桃炎です。この薬を飲んで、1日4回うがいをしてください。
You have tonsillitis. Take this medicine and gargle four times a day.

⑭のどが痛みますか。
Does your throat hurt?

⑮できるだけ声を使わないようにして、たばこはやめてください。
Use your voice as little as possible and give up smoking.

⑯自分でネブライザー療法(吸入療法)を行ってください。
You should treat yourself with the nebulizer.

⑰どちらの耳も同じように聞こえますか。
Do you hear the same in both ears?

⑱音叉を当てます。この音が聞こえなくなったら教えてください。
I am going to put this tuning fork here. Please tell me when you can no longer hear the sound.

⑲補聴器をつけていますか。
Do you wear a hearing aid?

⑳いつも大きな音や騒音にさらされていますか。
Are you regularly exposed to loud sounds or noise?

㉑左耳に耳鳴りがしますか。
Do you have ringing in your left ear?

㉒においはよくわかりますか。
Can you smell things?

㉓どのような鼻の病気にかかりましたか、鼻アレルギー、花粉症、それとも副鼻腔炎ですか。
What kind of nose problems have you experienced, nasal allergies, hay fever, or sinusitis?

患者さんからの表現例　**耳，鼻，咽喉，眼**

□耳がふさがった感じです。
　I feel as if my ears are blocked up.

□高音が聞こえにくいようなんです。
　I seem to have difficulty hearing high-pitched sounds.

□とても不快なので，喉頭炎ではないかと思います。
　I feel really bad, so I'm afraid I have laryngitis.

□この数カ月，声がかれています。
　For the past few months I've been hoarse.

⑨ Skin：皮膚

①ご使用の化粧品や香水に気をつけてください。
　Be careful about the cosmetics or perfumes you use.

②はしか，風疹，水疱瘡，手足口病は感染性発疹疾患です。
　Measles, rubella, chicken pox, hand-foot-mouth diseases are all infectious eruptive diseases.

③皮膚は脂っぽいですか，それとも乾燥してザラザラしていますか。
　Is your skin oily, or dry and rough?

④皮膚の色が，黒ずんだり，赤みを帯びたり，あるいは黄色っぽくなりましたか。
　Has your skin changed color, darker, reddish, or yellowish?

⑤他になにか皮膚に問題はありますか。
　Do you have any other skin problems?

患者さんからの表現例 皮膚

□腕に赤い(水疱状の)発疹があります。
I have a red (blistery) rash on my arms.

□ひどくかゆくて,痛いときもあります
It is very itchy and sometimes painful.

□顔のほくろが大きくなっています。
I'm afraid the mole on my face is getting bigger.

□放射線治療後,ひどい脱毛に悩んでいます。
After the radiation therapy, I am suffering from excessive hair loss.

⑩ Dentistry：歯科

①歯垢を取ります。
Let me remove the plaque from your teeth.

②歯のレントゲンをとります。
We are going to take an X-ray of your teeth.

③口を開けたままにしてください。
Keep your mouth open.

④歯を削って詰め物をします。
We will drill your tooth and fill it.

⑤このシートを2〜3回噛んでください。
Please bite on this sheet a couple of times.

⑥乳歯を抜かなければなりません。
We have to pull your baby tooth.

⑦口をゆすいでください。
Please rinse your mouth.

⑧冷たい飲み物が歯にしみますか。
Are your teeth sensitive when you have a cold drink?

⑨もう少し丁寧に歯を磨いてください。
You should brush your teeth more carefully.

⑩歯科衛生士がよい磨き方をみせてくれます。
The dental hygienist will show you how to brush your teeth well.

⑪麻酔が切れてから食べてください。
Please don't eat until the numbness has worn off.

⑪ Endocrine System：内分泌系

①甲状腺の病気と診断されたことがありますか。
Have you ever been diagnosed with thyroid disease?

②最近体重が増加あるいは減少しましたか。
Have you gained weight or lost weight recently?

③何回夜中に起きてトイレに行きますか。
How many times do you wake up to go to the bathroom at night?

④食欲はいかがですか。
How is your appetite?

⑤口の乾きに伴う他の徴候や症状はありますか。
Do you have any other signs or symptoms, accompanying by your dry mouth?

⑥抗うつ剤, あるいは抗ヒスタミン薬を常用していますか。
Are you taking any drugs such as antidepressants, or antihistamines?

身体の内部

⑫ Blood and Immune System：血液，免疫系

①顔が青白いですね。よく立ちくらみがありますか。
You look pale. Do you often feel dizzy when you stand up?

②貧血気味のようですね。寝汗はかきますか。
You seem to be anemic. Do you have night sweats?

③月経の変化に気づいていましたか。
Have you noticed any change in your〔menstrual〕periods?

④血液検査の結果を確認します。
Let me check your blood test results.

⑤出血しやすいですか。
Do you bleed easily?

⑥皮下出血を起こしやすいですか。
Do you bruise easily?

⑦出血が止まらないような経験がありますか。
Have you ever had bleeding that wouldn't stop?

⑧手術の後，輸血をしましたか。
Did you have a blood transfusion after the surgery?

患者さんからの表現例　血液，免疫系

□倦怠感や息切れも感じます。
I also feel fatigue and shortness of breath.

Symptoms

症候と徴候

Words and Terms 基本用語

① General Symptoms：一般的な症候

#		
1	☐ **pain; ache**	痛み
2	☐ itching; pruritus	かゆみ
3	☐ fever	熱
4	☐ **high fever (respirations;**	熱（呼吸数，脈拍など）が高い状
5	**pulse; etc.) ; pyrexia**	態
6	☐ chills	寒け，冷え，悪寒
7	☐ cough / coughing fits	咳／咳の発作
8	☐ **sore throat**	**喉の痛み**
9	☐ runny nose	鼻水
10	☐ nausea	悪心，吐き気
11	☐ poisoning; intoxication	中毒
12	☐ vomiting; emesis	嘔吐
13	☐ **dizziness**	めまい
14	☐ headache	頭痛
15	☐ **convulsion; paroxysm**	けいれん，ひきつけ，発作
16	☐ cyanosis	チアノーゼ
17	☐ dehydration	脱水症状
18	☐ shivering	ふるえ
19	☐ soreness	ひりひりすること
20	☐ stiffness	こり，硬直
21	☐ confusion	混乱
22	☐ **weakness**	**虚弱**

1	☐ slurred speech	不明瞭な話し方をすること
2	☐ stutter	どもり, 吃音
3	☐ 'not myself'	〔麻酔から覚めたときの様な〕自分でないような状態
5	☐ loss of energy (appetite; interest in sex)	エネルギー(食欲, 性欲)の喪失
7	☐ excessive appetite	食欲亢進
8	☐ **obesity**	**肥満**
9	☐ irritability	不機嫌
10	☐ **bleeding; hemorrhage**	**出血**
11	☐ feeling of fatigue	疲労感
12	☐ get tired easily	疲れやすいこと
13	☐ emaciation	るいそう, 異常なやせ細り
14	☐ **feeling of weariness**	**脱力感**
15	☐ hangover	二日酔い
16	☐ cold sweat	冷や汗
17	☐ night sweat	寝汗
18	☐ discharge	分泌物
19	☐ hot flash	体のほてり, のぼせ
20	☐ dry mouth	口唇が乾いていること
21	☐ dry throat	喉の乾き
22	☐ jaundice	黄疸
23	☐ edema	浮腫
24	☐ swelling	腫れ
25	☐ **polyp**	**ポリープ**
26	☐ rigidity	硬直
27	☐ bee sting	蜂刺され
28	☐ mosquito bite	蚊に刺されたあと
29	☐ episode	症状の発現, 発作
30	☐ anorexia	食欲不振

② Bone, Muscle, Joint：骨，筋，関節

- **stiff shoulder** — 肩こり
- backache — 背中の痛み
- **lumbago** — **腰痛**
- slipped disk — ぎっくり腰
- muscle pain — 筋肉痛
- muscle spasm — 筋肉のけいれん
- joint pain — 関節痛
- jammed finger — 突き指

③ Brain and Nervous System：脳，神経系

- irritability — いらいらしていること
- mood swings — 気分がゆれていること
- uneasiness; jitteriness — 落ち着かないこと, 神経過敏
- **anxiety** — **不安**
- ataxia — 運動失調
- aphasia — 失語
- migraine — 偏頭痛
- heaviness of the head — 頭が重い感じ
- **faint〔ness〕** — **気が遠くなる**（衰弱,失神,気絶）
- **memory loss** — **物忘れ**
- absent-mindedness — 放心〔状態〕
- **hallucination** — 〔一時的な〕**幻覚**
- auditory hallucination — 幻聴
- disorientation — 方向感覚を失うこと
- **paralysis** — **麻痺**
- **numbness** — **しびれ感**
- frustration — 欲求不満, フラストレーション
- nervousness — 緊張感

1	agitation	動揺, 興奮
2	**tension**	**緊張**
3	timidity	臆病
4	feeling of helplessness	無力感
5	hopelessness	絶望
6	delirium	狂乱, せん妄〔状態〕
7	coma	昏睡
8	tremor	振せん, 震え
9	vertigo	めまい

④ Respiratory System：呼吸器系

12	**mucus**	**粘液**
13	sneeze	くしゃみ
14	**sputum**	**痰**
15	phlegm	粘液分泌過多
16	hemoptysis	喀血
17	hoarseness	嗄声(させい)
18	breathing difficulty; dyspnea	呼吸困難
20	wheezing	ぜいぜい息をすること
21	shadow[S]	陰影
22	Cheyne-Strokes respiration	チェーンストークス呼吸, 交代性無呼吸
24	rale, crackle	ラ音, 水泡音

⑤ Circulatory System：循環器系

27	**palpitation**	**動悸**
28	**chest pain[CP]**	**胸痛**
29	feeling of pressure in one's chest	胸の圧迫感

1. ☐ **high blood pressure** 高血圧
2. **[HBP]; hypertension**
3. ☐ **low blood pressure** 低血圧
4. **[LBP]; hypotension**
5. ☐ rapid pulse; tachycardia 頻脈
6. ☐ slow pulse; bradycardia 徐脈
7. ☐ irregular pulse; 不整脈
8. arrhythmia
9. ☐ congestion うっ血

⑥ Digestive System：消化器系

12. ☐ **diarrhea** 下痢
13. ☐ **constipation** 便秘
14. ☐ **stomachache** 胃痛
15. ☐ burp げっぷ
16. ☐ vomiting blood 吐血
17. ☐ heartburn 胸やけ
18. ☐ epigastric distress 胃部不快感
19. ☐ sensation of stomach 胃圧迫感
20. pressure
21. ☐ heavy feeling in the 胃もたれ感
22. stomach
23. ☐ **loss of appetite** **食欲減退**
24. ☐ **abdominal pain** **腹痛**
25. ☐ bloating おなかがはること
26. ☐ abnormal bowel sounds 異常腸音
27. ☐ bloody stool 血便
28. ☐ loose bowel movement ゆるい便通
29. [s]

⑦ Kidney and Urinary System:腎・泌尿器系

- difficulty in urinating 排尿困難
- frequent urination 頻尿
- excessive urination; polyurina 多尿
- oliguria 乏尿
- anuria 無尿
- painful urination 痛みを伴う尿排泄
- bloody urine; hematuria 血尿
- glucosuria 糖尿
- **incontinence** 失禁
- urinary urgency 尿意促迫
- stress incontinence ストレス性失禁
- hematuria 血尿

⑧ Ear, Nose, Throat and Eye:耳,鼻,咽喉,眼

- ringing in one's ears 耳鳴り
- **difficulty in hearing** **難聴**
- ear pain 耳痛
- **earwax** **耳あか**
- ear discharge 耳漏(じろう)
- **nosebleed** **鼻血**
- nasal discharge 鼻水
- blocked nose; stuffy nose 鼻詰まり
- pain in the nose 鼻痛
- eye pain 眼痛
- **dry eye** **ドライアイ**
- teary eye; runny eye 涙目
- bloodshot eyes; red eyes 充血した目

1	☐ eye irritation	目がヒリヒリすること
2	☐ blurred vision	視覚のぼけ
3	☐ itchy eyes	目のかゆみ
4	☐ **eye mucus; eye matter**	**目やに**
5	☐ pus	膿
6	☐ dilation of the pupil	瞳孔散大
7	☐ photosensitivity	光過敏症

⑨ Skin：皮膚

10	☐ soft	やわらかい
11	☐ dry	乾燥した
12	☐ wet	湿気のある, 湿潤な
13	☐ **blistered**	**水ぶくれ(水疱)のある**
14	☐ **flushed**	**ほてり(熱感)のある**
15	☐ pale	蒼白な
16	☐ red; reddened	赤らんで, 顔面が紅潮した
17	☐ mottled	まだらの
18	☐ scaly	うろこ状の
19	☐ warm	ぽかぽかしている
20	☐ cool	ひんやりしている
21	☐ hot	熱い
22	☐ blanched	白っぽい
23	☐ **cracked**	**ひび割れた**
24	☐ excoriated; scraped	すりむいた, 傷ついた
25	☐ rough	ザラザラした, 粗い
26	☐ itch	かゆみ
27	☐ skin roughness	肌荒れ
28	☐ dry skin	乾燥肌
29	☐ skin eruption	皮疹
30	☐ **acne**	**にきび, 瘡**

1	☐ crust	かさぶた
2	☐ freckle	そばかす, しみ
3	☐ **mole**	**ほくろ, あざ**
4	☐ boil	おでき
5	☐ **rash; exanthema**	**発疹**
6	☐ **eczema**	**湿疹**
7	☐ roseola	バラ疹
8	☐ miliaria; heat rash	あせも, 汗疹
9	☐ hives; urticaria	じんましん
10	☐ goose bumps	鳥肌
11	☐ wrinkle; line	しわ
12	☐ lump	こぶ
13	☐ scar	傷跡, やけど跡
14	☐ **bedsore; decubitus ulcer**	**床ずれ, 褥瘡**
15	☐ blister	靴ずれ
16	☐ dandruff	ふけ
17	☐ baldness	はげ〔頭〕
18	☐ body odor	体臭

⑩ **Dentistry**:歯科

21	☐ mouth ulcer; canker sore	口内炎
22	☐ bad breath	口臭
23	☐ **saliva**	**唾液**
24	☐ **toothache**	**歯痛**
25	☐ **plaque**	**歯垢**
26	☐ twinge	〔歯痛などの〕激痛

⑪ Frequency：症状の頻度

- never — 決して〜ない
- **seldom** — めったに〜ない
- sometimes — ときどき
- occasionally — ときどき(sometimesより低い頻度)
- **frequently** — しばしば
- always — 常に
- sporadic — 散発性の, ときどき起こる
- episodic — 時折起こる
- **persistent; continuous** — **持続性の**
- reversible — 可逆性の
- irreversible — 不可逆性の
- **chronic** — **慢性の**
- **acute** — **急性の**
- recurring — 断続的な

⑫ Intensity：症状の強さ

- **slight** — わずかな, 軽微な, 軽い
- **mild** — 軽度の
- **moderate** — 中程度の
- **intense** — 激しい
- severe — 重篤な, 厳しい
- intolerable / barely tolerable — 我慢できない／なんとか我慢できる
- bearable / unbearable — 耐えうる／耐え難い
- intractable — 手に負えない, 治りにくい
- **severe pain** — ひどい痛み
- **sharp pain** — 激しい痛み

⑬ Types of Pain：痛みの種類

prickling pain	ちくちく刺すような痛み
stinging pain	刺痛
griping pain	きりきり(しくしく)する痛み
throbbing pain	ずきずきする痛み
squeezing pain	ギューッという痛み
crampy pain	差し込むような痛み, 疝痛
burning pain	焼けるような痛み
dull pain	鈍痛
slight pain	ちょっとした痛み
mild pain	軽い痛み
localized pain	局部的な痛み
generalized pain	全身の痛み
soreness	〔心身の〕うずき
gnawing pain	激痛
stitch	激痛, さしこみ

Expressions 表現

① 健康上の習慣：Health Habits

①たばこを吸いますか。
Do you smoke?

②1日に何本くらいたばこを吸いますか。
How many cigarettes do you smoke per day?

③お酒は飲みますか。
Do you drink alcohol?

④1日にどのくらいお酒を飲みますか。
How much alcohol do you drink in a day?

⑤食欲はありますか。
Do you have an appetite?
How is your appetite?

⑥食べられないものはありますか。
Are there any foods you cannot eat?

⑦菜食主義者ですか。
Are you a vegetarian?

⑧食べ物に対するアレルギーはありますか。
Are you allergic to any food?

⑨よく眠れますか。
Can you sleep well?
How is your sleep?

⑩毎日睡眠は何時間とっていますか。
How many hours do you sleep every night?

⑪夜中にどのくらいよく目が覚めますか？
How often do you wake up during the night?

⑫定期的にスポーツをしていますか。
Do you play any sports regularly?

患者さんからの表現例 健康上の習慣

☐ 1日に20本たばこを吸います。
  I smoke 20 cigarettes a day.

☐ 最近ほとんど食欲がありません。
  I don't have much of an appetite lately.

☐ 食後吐き気がします。
  I feel nauseated after meals.

☐ 血の混じったものを吐きました。
  I threw up a bloody mixture.

☐ 食後胃がもたれます。
  My stomach feels heavy after I eat.

☐ 胸焼けがします。
  I have heartburn.

☐ げっぷがよくでます。
  I burp a lot.

☐ 鶏肉アレルギーです。
  I am allergic to chickens.

☐ 毎日の睡眠時間は5時間ぐらいです。
  I sleep 5 hours a night.

② 排泄，生理：Excretion, Menstrual Period

①おしっこは1日何回ぐらいしますか。
How many times do you urinate per day?

②毎回おしっこの量はどのくらいですか。
How much do you urinate each time?

③おしっこのとき痛みますか。
Does it hurt when you urinate?

④規則正しい便通がありますか。頻度はどうですか？
Do you have regular bowel movements? How often?

⑤生理は順調ですか。
Are your periods regular?

患者さんからの表現例 排泄，生理

☐ 毎日下痢です。
I have diarrhea every day.

☐ 便秘です。
I am constipated.

☐ 血尿が出ます。
I have bloody urine.

☐ 生理中です。
I'm having my period.

☐ おりものが出ます。
I have a discharge.

☐ 夜中に何度もトイレに行かなければなりません。
I have to go to the toilet many times during the night.

3-04
Diseases, Conditions and Wounds
疾患と創傷

Words and Terms　基本用語

① Bone, Muscle, Joint：骨，筋，関節

1. ☐ **fracture**［fx］　　　　　　　骨折
2. ☐ osteoporosis　　　　　　　骨粗しょう症
3. ☐ **dislocation**　　　　　　　脱臼
4. ☐ **sprain**　　　　　　　ねんざ
5. ☐ cramp　　　　　　　けいれん
6. ☐ **arthritis**　　　　　　　**関節炎**
7. ☐ tendovaginitis;　　　　　　　腱鞘炎
8. 　tenosynovitis
9. ☐ rheumatism　　　　　　　リウマチ
10. ☐ rheumatoid arthritis［RA］　関節リウマチ
11. ☐ frozen shoulder　　　　　　　五十肩
12. ☐ whiplash injury　　　　　　　むち打ち症

② Brain and Nervous System：脳，神経系

15. ☐ **stroke**　　　　　　　脳卒中
16. ☐ **cerebral infarction**　　　　　　　**脳梗塞**
17. ☐ cerebral thrombosis　　　　　　　脳血栓症
18. ☐ subarachnoid　　　　　　　くも膜下出血
19. 　hemorrhage［SAH］
20. ☐ intracerebral hemorrhage　　脳〔内〕出血

1	☐ transient ischemic attack [TIA]	一過性脳虚血発作
3	☐ **brain tumor**	**脳腫瘍**
4	☐ brain concussion	脳しんとう〔症〕
5	☐ cerebral anemia	脳貧血
6	☐ epilepsy	てんかん
7	☐ **neuralgia**	**神経痛**
8	☐ facial neuralgia	顔面神経痛
9	☐ hemiplegia	片(半側)麻痺
10	☐ photophobia	光恐怖〔症〕
11	☐ photosensitivity	光過敏性

③ Respiratory System：呼吸器系

14	☐ pneumonia	肺炎
15	☐ lung cancer	肺がん
16	☐ pulmonary emphysema	肺気腫
17	☐ **tuberculosis [TB]**	**結核**
18	☐ bronchitis	気管支炎
19	☐ **asthma**	**喘息**
20	☐ pneumothorax	気胸

④ Circulatory System：循環器系

23	☐ coronary artery disease	冠状動脈疾患
24	☐ heart disease	心臓病
25	☐ **heart attack**	**心臓発作**
26	☐ **heart failure**	**心不全**
27	☐ myocardial infarction [MI]	心筋梗塞
28	☐ cardiomyopathy	心筋症
29	☐ myocarditis	心筋炎
30	☐ **angina [pectoris]**	**狭心症**

1	☐ aortic aneurysm	大動脈瘤
2	☐ arrhythmia	不整脈

⑤ Digestive System：消化器系

5	☐ **gastritis**	**胃炎**
6	☐ gastric ulcer［GU］	胃潰瘍
7	☐ stomach cramp	胃けいれん
8	☐ duodenal ulcer［DU］	十二指腸潰瘍
9	☐ pancreatitis	膵炎
10	☐ **hepatitis**	**肝炎**
11	☐ liver cirrhosis	肝硬変
12	☐ liver cancer; hepatic cancer	肝臓がん
14	☐ cholecystitis	胆のう炎
15	☐ gallstones	胆石〔症〕
16	☐ **bile duct calculus**	**胆管結石**
17	☐ enteritis	腸炎
18	☐ **colon cancer**	**大腸がん**
19	☐ colitis	大腸炎
20	☐ intestinal obstruction	腸閉塞
21	☐ volvulus	腸捻転(ちょうねんてん)
22	☐ **appendicitis**	**虫垂炎(盲腸炎)**
23	☐ peritonitis	腹膜炎
24	☐ rectal cancer	直腸がん
25	☐ food poisoning	食中毒
26	☐ **diarrhea**	**下痢**

⑥ Kidney and Urinary System：腎・泌尿器系

29	☐ cystitis	膀胱炎
30	☐ **nephritis**	**腎炎**

1	☐ pyelitis	腎盂炎
2	☐ nephrosis	ネフローゼ
3	☐ kidney failure	腎不全
4	☐ prostate cancer	前立腺がん
5	☐ urinary stone	尿路結石
6	☐ urinary tract infection	尿路感染症
7	☐ pyuria	膿尿症
8	☐ albuminuria	蛋白尿〔症〕, アルブミン尿〔症〕
9	☐ anuria	無尿〔症〕
10	☐ choluria	胆汁尿〔症〕
11	☐ dysuria	排尿障害, 排尿困難
12	☐ nocturia	夜間多尿〔症〕
13	☐ oliguria	尿量過少, 乏尿〔症〕
14	☐ polyuria	多尿〔症〕
15	☐ pyuria	膿尿 (排尿時, 尿中に膿が存在すること)

⑦ Ear, Nose, Throat and Eye：耳, 鼻, 咽喉, 眼

19	☐ **otitis media**	**中耳炎**
20	☐ **tonsillitis**	**扁桃炎**
21	☐ **rhinitis**	**鼻炎**
22	☐ pollinosis; hay fever	花粉症
23	☐ **cataract[cat.]**	**白内障**
24	☐ glaucoma	緑内障
25	☐ trachoma	トラコーマ
26	☐ macular degeneration	黄斑変性
27	☐ astigmatism	乱視
28	☐ amblyopia	弱視
29	☐ retinopathy	網膜症, 網膜障害

#		
1	☐ sty	ものもらい
2	☐ **blindness**	**失明**
3	☐ keratitis	角膜炎
4	☐ conjunctivitis	結膜炎
5	☐ diplopia	複視, 二重視(単一の物体が2個
6		の物体に見える状態)
7	☐ mydriasis	散瞳, 瞳孔散大
8	☐ **myopia**	**近視**
9	☐ myosis	縮瞳
10	☐ strabismus	斜視

⑧ Skin：皮膚

#		
13	☐ **cut**	**切り傷**
14	☐ contusion	打撲症, 挫傷
15	☐ **bite**	**かまれた跡, 刺し傷**
16	☐ stab	刺し傷
17	☐ scratch; abrasion	すり傷
18	☐ bruise	打撲傷
19	☐ laceration	裂傷
20	☐ bump; lump	こぶ, たんこぶ
21	☐ abraded wound	擦過創
22	☐ excoriation; scrape	すり傷, 擦〔過〕創, 爪痕
23	☐ skin cancer	皮膚がん
24	☐ **atopic dermatitis**	**アトピー性皮膚炎**
25	☐ dry skin	乾皮症(かんぴしょう)
26	☐ **burn**	**やけど, 熱傷**
27	☐ melanoma	メラノーマ, 黒色腫
28	☐ alopecia	脱毛症
29	☐ **athlete's foot**	**水虫**
30	☐ hircismus; body odor	わきが

1	☐ **wart**	いぼ
2	☐ chap	ひび, あかぎれ
3	☐ clavus	うおのめ
4	☐ urticaria	じんましん

⑨ Dentistry：歯科

7	☐ **decayed tooth; cavity;**	虫歯
8	**dental caries**	
9	☐ pyorrhea	歯槽膿漏症
10	☐ tartar	歯石

⑩ Endocrine System：内分泌系

13	☐ gout	痛風
14	☐ **diabetes**	**糖尿病**
15	☐ Basedow's disease	バセドー氏病
16	☐ Hashimoto thyroiditis	橋本甲状腺炎
17	☐ Cushing's disease	クッシング病

⑪ Blood and Immune System：血液, 免疫系

20	☐ **anemia**	**貧血**
21	☐ **leukemia**	**白血病**
22	☐ hemophilia	血友病
23	☐ malignant lymphoma	悪性リンパ腫
24	☐ collagenosis	膠原病
25	☐ immunocompromised	免疫無防備状態

⑫ Infectious Diseases：感染症

28	☐ **flu; influenza**	インフルエンザ
29	☐ malaria	マラリア
30	☐ **cholera**	コレラ

1	☐ severe acute respiratory	重症急性呼吸器症候群
2	syndrome [SARS]	
3	☐ **acquired**	エイズ
4	**immunodeficiency**	
5	**syndrome [AIDS]**	
6	☐ human	HIVウイルス
7	immunodeficiency virus	
8	[HIV]	
9	☐ **sexually transmitted**	**性感染症**
10	**disease [STD]**	
11	☐ gonorrhea	淋病
12	☐ syphilis	梅毒
13	☐ **herpes**	**疱疹, ヘルペス**
14	☐ hepatitis	肝炎
15	☐ dengue fever	デング熱
16	☐ gastroenteritis	〔急性感染性〕胃腸炎
17	☐ **Norovirus**	**ノロウイルス**
18	☐ viral hepatitis	ウイルス性肝炎
19	☐ **avian flu**	**鳥インフルエンザ**
20	☐ swine flu	豚インフルエンザ
21	☐ parrot fever	オウム病
22	☐ rabies	狂犬病
23	☐ Ebola hemorrhagic fever	エボラ出血熱
24	☐ West Nile fever	西ナイル熱

Expressions 表現

①以前に何か大きな病気をしたことがありますか。
Have you ever had a serious illness?

②入院したことがありますか。
Have you ever been hospitalized?

③手術を受けたことがありますか。
Have you ever had any surgery?

④ご家族に同じ病気の方はおられますか。
Is there anyone in your family who has (had) the same illness?

⑤ご両親は何か大きな病気をされたことがありますか。
Do your parents have any serious medical problems?

⑥何か常用している薬はありますか。
Are you taking any medication regularly?
What medicines do you take (use) regularly?

患者さんからの表現例　手術，薬，病状

□5年前乳がんになりました。
I had breast cancer 5 years ago.

□子供のとき手術を受けました。
I had an operation when I was a child.

□この薬は効きません。
This medicine doesn't work.

Diagnostic Tests
検査

Words and Terms 基本用語

① Common Tests：一般的な検査

physical examination (checkup)	身体検査
blood pressure[BP]	血圧
temperature	体温
ultrasonography[US]	超音波検査
biopsy[Bx]	生検
sputum examination	喀痰検査
X-ray examination[X-P]	X線検査
computerized axial tomography[CAT]	X線体軸断層撮影法
chest X-ray (radiograph)	胸部X線検査
screening study	スクリーニング検査
computerized tomography scan[CT]	CTスキャン
magnetic resonance imaging[MRI]	磁気共鳴画像法
positron emission tomography[PET]	ポジトロンCT, 陽電子放出断層撮影
physiological function test	生理学的機能検査
the subjective well-being inventory[SUBI]	主観的幸福感を見る尺度

3-05 Diagnostic Tests

1. ☐ stress test — ストレステスト
2. ☐ pathology examination — 病理検査
3. ☐ bacteria culture — 細菌検査
4. ☐ cytotechnology — 細胞検査
5. **DNA testing** — DNA 検査
6. ☐ genetic testing — 遺伝子検査
7. ☐ HIV antibody test — HIV 抗体テスト
8. ☐ immunological test — 免疫〔学的〕検査

② Bone, Muscle, Joint：骨，筋，関節

11. ☐ **electromyography [EMG]** — 筋電図検査
12. ☐ arthrography — 関節造影
13. ☐ rheumatoid arthritis test [RA test] — 関節リウマチ(RA)試験

③ Brain and Nervous System：脳，神経系

17. ☐ cerebrospinal fluid examination [CSF exam.] — 脳脊髄液検査
19. ☐ **electroencephalography [EEG]** — 脳波検査
21. ☐ myelography — 脊髄造影
22. ☐ **tendon reflex** — 腱反射

④ Respiratory System：呼吸器系

25. ☐ **pulmonary function test [PFT]** — 肺機能検査
27. ☐ spirometry — 肺活量測定検査
28. ☐ bronchoscopy — 気管支鏡検査
29. ☐ fiber bronchoscopy — ファイバー気管支鏡検査

検査

⑤ Circulatory System：循環器系

- **electrocardiogram[ECG; EKG]** 心電図
- **cardiac catheterization** **心臓カテーテル検査**
- phonocardiography 心音図検査
- angiocardiography 血管心臓造影
- angiography 血管造影
- aortography 大動脈造影
- cavography 大静脈造影
- **treadmill test** **トレッドミル試験**
- color Doppler echocardiography カラードップラー法による心エコー検査
- Doppler ultrasonography ドップラー超音波検査
- feces (stool) test 検便
- **endoscopic examination; endoscopy** 内視鏡検査
- laparoscopic examination; laparoscopy 腹腔鏡検査

⑥ Digestive System：消化器系

- esophagoscopy 食道鏡検査
- **gastroscopy** **胃カメラ検査**
- gastric analysis[GA] 胃液検査
- gastrofiberscopy 胃ファイバースコープ検査
- gastrointestinal endoscopy 胃腸内視鏡検査
- colonoscopy 大腸鏡検査
- barium enema[BE] バリウム注腸
- **liver function test[LFT]** **肝機能検査**

1	☐ hemoccult test	潜血試験
2	☐ test for ova; parasites	寄生虫の検査
3	☐ fiberoptic endoscopy	ファイバー内視鏡検査

⑦ Kidney and Urinary System：腎・泌尿器系

6	☐ **urine test; urinalysis[UA]**	尿検査
7	☐ renal function test	腎機能検査
8	☐ specific gravity[SG]	比重
9	☐ acetone	アセトン
10	☐ urobilinogen[U]	ウロビリノーゲン
11	☐ **ketone body**	**ケトン体**

⑧ Ear, Nose, Throat and Eye：耳，鼻，咽喉，眼

14	☐ ophthalmic examination	眼科検査
15	☐ examination of the fundus	眼底検査
17	☐ **eye test**	**視力検査**
18	☐ color perception test	色覚検査
19	☐ pupillary reflex	瞳孔反射
20	☐ examination of the visual field	視野検査
22	☐ intraocular pressure measurement	眼圧測定
24	☐ **hearing test**	**聴力検査**

⑨ Endocrine System：内分泌系

27	☐ fasting hypoglycemia	空腹時性低血糖
28	☐ **growth hormone[GH]**	**成長ホルモン**
29	☐ **thyroid-stimulating hormone[TSH]**	**甲状腺刺激ホルモン**

1	☐ **adrenocorticotropic hormone[ACTH]**	副腎皮質刺激ホルモン
3	☐ gonadotropic hormone[GTH]	性腺刺激ホルモン
5	☐ human chorionic gonadotropin[HCG; hCG]	ヒト絨毛性ゴナドトロピン
7	☐ prolactin[PRL]	プロラクチン
8	☐ antidiuretic hormone[ADH]	抗利尿ホルモン
10	☐ protein bound iodine[PBI]	蛋白結合ヨウ素
12	☐ aldosterone[ALD, Ald]	アルドステロン
13	☐ **glucose tolerance test[GTT]**	**ブドウ糖負荷試験**
15	☐ oral glucose tolerance test[OGTT]	経口ブドウ糖負荷試験
17	☐ prednisolone-glucose tolerance test[PGTT]	プレドニゾロン・ブドウ糖負荷試験
19	☐ cortisone-glucose tolerance test[CGTT]	コルチゾン・ブドウ糖負荷試験
21	☐ insulin sensitivity test	インスリン感受性試験
22	☐ **fasting blood sugar[FBS]**	**空腹時血糖**

⑩ Blood：血液

(a) general：一般

26	☐ blood sample	血液標本
27	☐ blood sugar test	血糖検査
28	☐ **blood type**	**血液型**
29	☐ blood volume[BV]	血液量

1	☐ complete blood count [CBC]	全血球計算値(全血算)
3	☐ biochemical examination of blood	生化学血液検査
5	☐ **blood plasma[BP]**	血漿
6	☐ **blood serum[BS]**	血清
7	☐ **red blood cell [RBC]; erythrocyte**	赤血球
9	☐ **white blood cell[WBC]; leukocyte**	白血球
11	☐ red blood count[RBC]	赤血球数
12	☐ serological test	血清検査
13	☐ blood platelet[Plat]	血小板
14	☐ hemoglobin[Hb]	血色素量(ヘモグロビン)
15	☐ hematocrit[Hct]	血球容量(ヘマトクリット値)
16	☐ blood sedimentation rate [BSR; SED rate]	赤血球沈降速度
18	☐ **sodium[Na]**	ナトリウム
19	☐ potassium; kalium[K]	カリウム
20	☐ chloride[Cl]	塩素
21	☐ **calcium[Ca]**	カルシウム
22	☐ magnesium[Mg]	マグネシウム
23	☐ glucose[Glu]	ブドウ糖
24	☐ total protein[TP]	総蛋白
25	☐ albumin[Alb]	アルブミン
26	☐ globulin[Glob]	グロブリン
27	☐ **albumin-globulin ratio [A/G ratio]**	アルブミン・グロブリン比
29	☐ ammonia[NH3]	アンモニア
30	☐ urea nitrogen[Urea-N]	尿素窒素

1	☐ **creatinine [Crea]**	クレアチニン
2	☐ uric acid [UA]	尿酸
3	☐ **total cholesterol [TC]**	**総コレステロール**
4	☐ triglyceride [TG]	トリグリセリド(中性脂肪)
5	☐ fatty acid [FA]	脂肪酸
6	☐ free fatty acid [FFA]	遊離脂肪酸
7	☐ ferrum [Fe]	鉄
8	☐ phospholipid [PL]	リン脂質
9	☐ total bilirubin [TBil]	総ビリルビン
10	☐ direct bilirubin [DBil]	直接型ビリルビン

(b) blood clotting：血液凝固

12	☐ **fibrinogen [Fbg]**	**フィブリノーゲン**
13	☐ prothrombin time [PT]	プロトロンビン時間
14-15	☐ partial thromboplastin time [PTT]	部分トロンボプラスチン時間
16	☐ bleeding time [BT]	出血時間
17	☐ **coagulation time [CT]**	**凝固時間**
18-20	☐ activated partial thromboplastin time [aPTT]	活性化部分トロンボプラスチン時間
21	☐ thrombo test [TBT]	トロンボテスト
22	☐ thrombin time [TT]	トロンビン時間
23-24	☐ tissue thromboplastin inhabitation test [TTIT]	トロンボプラスチン抑制試験
25-27	☐ fibrin and fibrinogen degradation product [FDP]	フィブリン分解産物

⑪ Equipment and Supplies：検査機器

- **spirometer** 肺活量計
- bronchoscope 気管支鏡
- **gastrocamera** 胃カメラ
- fiberscope ファイバースコープ
- **endoscope** 内視鏡
- proctoscope 直腸鏡
- Holter monitor ホルター心電計
- **stethoscope** 聴診器
- hand dynamometer 握力計
- cup 〔尿検査用〕コップ
- container 容器(検便用)
- glass stick 〔検便用〕ガラス棒
- **audiometer** 聴力計
- catheter カテーテル
- eye chart 視力検査表
- gauge 計測器
- laparoscope 腹腔鏡
- **microscope** 顕微鏡
- electron microscope 電子顕微鏡
- ophthalmoscope 検眼鏡
- protective shield; lead apron 放射線用プロテクター
- **tuning fork** 音叉
- X-ray apparatus X線撮影装置
- contrast medium 造影剤

Expressions 表現

① Blood Test：血液検査

①血液検査をしますが、今よろしいですか。
I need to take a blood sample for testing. May I do it now?

②左手を出してください。
Please hold out your left arm.

③握りこぶしを作ってください。
Please make a fist.

④チクッとしますよ。
This may hurt a little.

⑤どうぞ楽にして、深呼吸をしてください。
Please relax. Breathe in and out slowly and deeply.

② Collecting Urine and Stool Specimens：尿検査，便検査

①尿検査をさせてください。
Please help me by filling this cup for a urine test.

②尿が出ますか。
Can you urinate?

③最初の尿は捨てて、カップの1/3ぐらいまで尿を入れてください。
Please throw away the first urine, then fill the cup about one-third full with urine.

④明日朝起きたら、このコップの1/3まで尿をとってください。
Please collect a third cup from your first urination tomorrow morning.

⑤尿を入れたカップはトイレの棚に置いてください。
Leave the cup of urine on the shelf in the toilet.

⑥検便をさせてください。
We need to test your stool.

 患者さんからの表現例 **尿検査，便検査**

□尿(便)はどのぐらいとるのですか。
How much urine (stool) should I collect?

③ EKG, etc. : 心電図など

①心電図(X線写真, CTスキャン, MRI, PET)を撮る準備をしてください。
Let's get ready to go for your EKG (X-ray, CT, MRI, PET).

②もうすぐMRIの時間です。
It's almost time for your MRI.

③医師からCTスキャンを行うよう指示を受けました。
The doctor has ordered a CT.

患者さんからの表現例 心電図など

☐ 1年前に心電図をとりました。
I had an EKG a year ago.

☐ 下着は着ていてもいいですか。
Can I keep my underwear on?

☐ このガウンに着替えるのですか。
Should I change into the gown?

☐ 衣服はどこに入れればいいですか。
Where should I put my clothes?

☐ 検査はどのぐらいの時間かかるのですか。
How long does it take to finish this test?

☐ 検査中眠っていいですか。
Can I sleep during the test?

☐ 検査の結果はいつわかりますか。
When will I get the results of the test?

☐ 精密検査を受けなければなりませんか。
Will I need a follow-up examination?

Physical Examination

診察

Words and Terms　基本用語

① General Terms：一般用語

1. ☐ present condition　現症
2. ☐ **symptom**　症状
3. ☐ **sign**　徴候
4. ☐ **syndrome**　症候群
5. ☐ number; numero [No]　番号
6. ☐ **inspection; palpitation; percussion; auscultation [IPPA]**　視診, 触診, 打診, 聴診
9. ☐ general status　全身状態
10. ☐ anisocoria　瞳孔不同
11. ☐ location　位置
12. ☐ oblique [OB]　斜位の
13. ☐ superior [sup]　上方の
14. ☐ inferior [inf]　下方の
15. ☐ lateral [lat]　側方の
16. ☐ internal [int]　内の
17. ☐ external [ext]　外の
18. ☐ right [R]; dexter [d.; dext]　右の
19. ☐ left [L]; sinister [s.; sin]　左の
20. ☐ accommodation [A]　調節
21. ☐ nothing particular; no problem [np]　異常なし

1	☐ slightly [SL]	わずかに
2	☐ positive [Pos]	陽性
3	☐ negative [Neg]	陰性
4	☐ adduction [add]	内転
5	☐ abduction [abd]	外転

② Vital Signs：バイタルサイン

8	☐ blood pressure [BP]	血圧
9	☐ body temperature [BT]	体温
10	☐ **centigrade (Celsius) [°C]**	摂氏度
11	☐ **Fahrenheit [°F]**	華氏度
12	☐ high fever	高熱
13	☐ slight fever	微熱
14	☐ intermittent fever	間欠熱
15	☐ remittent fever	弛張熱
16	☐ **bradycardia [bra]; slow pulse**	徐脈
18	☐ **tachycardia**	頻脈
19	☐ quick pulse	速脈
20	☐ arrhythmia	不整脈
21	☐ **apnea**	**無呼吸**
22	☐ hyperpnea	過呼吸
23	☐ **pulse [P]**	**脈拍**
24	☐ chest	胸部
25	☐ cardiorespiratory [CR]	心呼吸系
26	☐ hyperventilation	過換気
27	☐ hypoventilation	低換気
28	☐ anoxia	無酸素症
29	☐ **systolic blood pressure [SBP]**	収縮期血圧

- [ ] **diastolic blood pressure [DBP]** 拡張期血圧
- [ ] mean blood pressure [MBP] 平均血圧
- [ ] hypoxia 低酸素血症
- [ ] **heart rate [HR]** **心拍数**
- [ ] respiration [R] 呼吸
- [ ] respiratory rate [RR] 呼吸数

③ Physical Check-up：健康診断

- [ ] **height [Ht]** **身長**
- [ ] **weight [Wt]** **体重**
- [ ] head circumference [HC] 頭囲
- [ ] chest circumference [CC] 胸囲
- [ ] abdominal circumference [AC] 腹囲
- [ ] body surface area [BSA] 体表面積
- [ ] gingiva [G] 歯肉
- [ ] body odor [BO] 体臭
- [ ] light sense [LS] 光覚
- [ ] visual acuity [VA] 視力
- [ ] visual field [VF] 視野
- [ ] eye ocular movement [EOM] 眼球運動
- [ ] artery [A] 動脈
- [ ] vein [V] 静脈
- [ ] pulse pressure [PP] 脈圧
- [ ] heart sound [HS] 心音
- [ ] cardiac murmur [m] 心雑音

1	breath sound[BS];	呼吸音
2	respiratory sound[RS]	
3	shortness of breath[SOB]	息切れ
4	intercostal [IC]	肋間の
5	mid line[ML]	正中
6	bowel sound[BS]	腸雑音
7	finger breadth[FB]	横指
8	bone and joint[B&J]	骨と関節
9	reflex[ref]	反射
10	Achilles' tendon reflex	アキレス腱反射
11	[ATR / ankle jerk; AJ]	
12	biceps jerk[BJ]	二頭筋反射
13	deep tendon reflex[DTR]	深部腱反射
14	patellar tendon reflex	膝蓋腱反射
15	[PTR]	
16	grasping power[GP]	握力
17	nerve[N]	神経
18	**cranial nerve[CN]**	**脳神経**
19	**cervical [C]**	頚椎の,頚髄の
20	**thoracic[Th]**	胸椎の,胸髄の
21	**lumbar[L]**	腰椎の,腰髄の
22	**sacral [S]**	仙骨の,仙髄の
23	hand motion[HM]	手動弁
24	counting fingers[CF]	指数弁
25	lymph node[LN]	リンパ節

Expressions 表現

① Blood Pressure：血圧

①血圧を計ります。
Let me take your blood pressure.

②袖をまくってください。
Roll up your sleeve please.

③ゆっくり息を吸って吐いてください。
Please breathe in and out slowly.

④血圧は140/75です。
Your blood pressure is 140 over 75.

⑤あなたの通常の血圧はどのくらいですか。
What is your usual blood pressure?

② Body Temperature：体温

①体温を計ります。
Let me take your temperature.

②タオルで汗をふいてください。
Please wipe away the sweat with this towel.

③3分間体温計をわきの下にはさんでおいてください。
You must keep the thermometer under your arm for 3 minutes.

④ピーという音が聞こえたら体温計を出してください。
Take out the thermometer when you hear the beeping sound.

Treatment and Therapy

治療と療法

Words and Terms 基本用語

① Treatment and Operations：治療と手術

1	☐ **emergency medical service [EMS]**	救急医療
3	☐ basic life support [BLS]	1次救命処置
4	☐ advanced life support [ALS]	2次救命処置
6	☐ intravenous (IV) injection	静脈注射
7	☐ subcutaneous injection	皮下注射
8	☐ intradermal injection	皮内注射
9	☐ intramuscular injection	筋肉注射
10	☐ **intravenous drip**	**点滴**
11	☐ **blood transfusion**	**輸血**
12	☐ hemostasis	止血
13	☐ **first aid**	**応急処置**
14	☐ artificial respiration	人工呼吸
15	☐ inhalation	吸入
16	☐ suction	吸引
17	☐ detoxication	解毒
18	☐ anesthesia	麻酔
19	☐ local anesthesia	局所麻酔
20	☐ general anesthesia	全身麻酔
21	☐ **surgery**	**手術**
22	☐ emergency surgery	緊急手術

1. **outpatient surgery** — 日帰り手術
2. palliative operation — 姑息的手術
3. radical operation — 根治手術
4. **living-donor operation** — 生体移植手術
5. organ transplantation — 臓器移植
6. cardiac surgery — 心臓手術
7. heart bypass operation — 心臓のバイパス手術
8. brain surgery — 脳外科手術
9. plastic surgery — 形成外科手術
10. **cosmetic surgery** — 美容整形
11. endoscopic operation — 内視鏡手術
12. laser surgery — レーザー手術
13. extirpative surgery — 摘出手術
14. lumpectomy — 腫瘍摘出手術
15. incision — 切開
16. suture — 縫合
17. intubation — 挿管
18. catheterization — カテーテル法
19. **dialysis** — 透析
20. hot (cold) compress — 温(冷)湿布
21. **enema [E]** — 浣腸
22. stool extraction — 摘便
23. **shaving hair** — 剃毛

② Therapies : 療法

26. **radiation therapy [RT]** — 放射線療法
27. oral rehydration therapy [ORT] — 経口輸液療法
29. symptomatic (control) therapy — 対症療法

治療と療法

1	☐ climatotherapy	気候療法
2	☐ surgical therapy	外科的治療
3	☐ medical therapy	内科的治療
4	☐ **drug therapy; medication**	**薬物治療**
5	☐ **chemotherapy**	**化学療法**
6	☐ gene therapy	遺伝子治療
7	☐ regenerative therapy	再生医療
8	☐ immune therapy	免疫療法
9	☐ hormone therapy	ホルモン療法
10	☐ **palliative treatment**	**緩和療法**
11	☐ diet therapy	食事療法
12	☐ speech therapy [ST]	言語療法
13	☐ alternative medicine	代替医療
14	☐ complementary therapy	相補療法
15	☐ physical therapy	理学療法
16	☐ thermal therapy	温熱治療
17	☐ treatment with hot baths	温浴療法
18	☐ spa therapy	温泉療法
19	☐ infrared therapy	赤外線療法
20	☐ light therapy	光線療法
21	☐ exercise therapy	運動療法
22	☐ massage therapy	マッサージ療法
23	☐ occupational therapy	作業療法
24	☐ horticulture therapy;	園芸療法
25	social and therapeutic	
26	horticulture [STH]	
27	☐ psychological therapy;	心理療法
28	mental therapy	
29	☐ hypnotic therapy	催眠療法
30	☐ cognitive therapy	認知療法

PART3 解剖・徴候・疾患の基本用語と表現

1	☐ sand play therapy	箱庭療法
2	☐ behavior therapy[BT]	行動療法
3	☐ play therapy	遊戯療法
4	☐ recreation therapy	レクリエーション療法
5	☐ health resort therapy	転地療法
6	☐ aroma therapy	アロマセラピー
7	☐ art therapy[AT]	芸術療法
8	☐ color therapy	色彩療法
9	☐ music therapy	音楽療法
10	☐ family therapy	家族療法
11	☐ group therapy	集団療法
12	☐ individual therapy	個人療法
13	☐ animal therapy	アニマルセラピー, 動物介在療法
15	☐ laughter therapy	笑い療法
16	☐ therapeutic touch	タッチ療法
17	☐ chronotherapy	時間治療
18	☐ herbal therapy	薬草療法
19-20	☐ **acupuncture and moxibustion therapy**	**鍼灸治療**
21	☐ homeopathy	ホメオパシー
22	☐ chiropractic	カイロプラクティック
23	☐ reflexology	リフレクソロジー
24	☐ energy-based therapy	エネルギー療法
25-26	☐ electroconvulsive therapy [TCT]	電気ショック療法
27	☐ radical treatment	根治療法
28	☐ (**cardiac**) pacemaker	心臓ペースメーカー

③ Posture, Position：体位

- standing position 立位
- sitting position 坐位
- recumbent position 臥位
- dorsal (supine) position; supination 仰臥(背臥)位
- dorsal recumbent position 背横位
- knee-chest position 膝胸位
- prone position 腹臥位
- lateral position 側臥位
- lithotomy position 切石位, 砕石位
- Trendelenburg's position トレンデレンブルグ体位
- Fowler's position ファウラー体位
- semi-Fowler position 半ファウラー体位
- Sims' position シムズ体位
- abduction 外転
- adduction 内転

Expressions 表現

① 注射,点滴:Injection, IV

①点滴を始めます。
I'll start the IV now.

②いまから点滴に抗生剤を追加します。
It is time now to add the antibiotic to your IV drip.

③注射をします。
I'll give you an injection (a shot).

④注射が痛かったり,赤くなってきたら言ってください。
Please tell me if the place around the needle begins to hurt or look red.

 患者さんからの表現例　注射,点滴

☐点滴はどのぐらい時間がかかりますか。
How long will it be until the IV is finished?

☐なぜ注射が必要なのですか。
Why do I need an injection?

☐針は安全ですか。
Is the needle safe?

☐少しの間なら我慢できます。
I can stand it for a little while.

② 包帯など：Bandage, etc.

①足に包帯をします。
I'll wrap this bandage around your leg.

②包帯を取り替えます。
I'm going to put a fresh dressing on your wound.

③包帯がきつかったら教えてください。
Please let me know if the bandage is too tight.

④傷の消毒をします。
I'll disinfect the wound.

⑤傷口を見せてください。
Show me your wound.

⑥傷口のまわりの毛を剃ります。
I'm going to shave away the hair around the wound.

⑦止血します。
I'll stop the bleeding.

⑧〜に湿布をします。
I'll put a compress on your... .

⑨浣腸をします。
I'm going to give you an enema.

⑩指で便を出します。
I'll try to remove the stool with my fingers.

患者さんからの表現例　包帯など

□包帯はいつ取り替えてもらえますか。
When will you change the bandage?

□包帯をしてお風呂に入っていいですか。
Can I take a bath with the bandage on?

③ 体位など：Body Position, etc.

①力を抜いて,ベッドに横になってください。
Please relax and lie down on the bed.

②診察台の上に腹ばいになってください。
Lie on your stomach on the examination table.

③仰向けに寝てください。
Lie on your back.

④左を下にして横になってください。
Lie on your left side.

⑤反対側を向いてください。
Turn over.

⑥仰向けに(うつ伏せに,横に)なってください。
Please roll over onto your back (stomach; side).

⑦(寝た状態から)上半身を起こしてください。
Sit up.

⑧左をむいてください。
Turn to the left.

⑨右手を出してください。
May I have your right hand?

⑩動かないでください。
Please don't move.

⑪足を伸ばしてください。
Stretch out your legs.

⑫足を上げてください。
Put your feet up.

⑬私の手を握ってください。
Hold my hand.

Index

あ

あかぎれ	152
赤ちゃん	13
赤ちゃん言葉	13
赤らんで	140
アキレス腱	117
アキレス腱反射	169
悪性の	7
悪性リンパ腫	152
アクセサリー	103
あくびをする	99
握力	169
握力計	162
顎	112
あざ	141
脚	114
——の付け根	113
足	114
——の裏	114
——の親指	114
——の小指	114
——の甲	114
足首	114
味付け	100
脚のせ	67
足指	114
——の爪	114
アセスメント	55
アセトン	158
あせも	13, 141
焦り	18
汗をかく	99
頭	112
——が重い感じ	136
アダルト・チルドレン	16
熱い	140
圧縮空気差込プラグ	67
圧迫帯	67
後産	23
アトピー性皮膚炎	11, 151
アニマルセラピー	174
アプガースコア	10, 13
油紙	65
粗い	140
アルコール依存	19
アルコール依存症	17
アルツハイマー病	38
アルドステロン	159
アルブミン	160
アルブミン・グロブリン比	160
アルブミン尿〔症〕	150
アレルギー	93
アレルギー反応	3
アレルゲン除去	12
アロマセラピー	174
安心感	39
案内係	63
アンモニア	160
安楽死	40
安楽のケア	42

い

胃	119
胃圧迫感	138
胃液	119
胃液検査	157
胃炎	149
胃潰瘍	149
胃カメラ	162
胃カメラ検査	157
怒り	19, 41
胃管	68
生きがい	39
息切れ	169
いきむ	23
育児相談	13
胃けいれん	149
医師	82
医師法	52
いじめ	34
異常腸音	138
異常なし	166
異常なやせ細り	135
依存症	16
痛み	134
——を伴う尿排泄	139
位置	166
一時的緩和	41
一時的保育サービス	35
胃腸炎	153
胃腸内視鏡検査	157
胃腸薬	95
胃痛	138

一過性脳虚血発作	148
一般開業医	82
一般病棟	62
遺伝	26
遺伝子検査	156
遺伝子治療	173
遺伝病	5
居眠りをする	99
胃ファイバースコープ検査	157
胃部不快感	138
いぼ	152
胃もたれ感	138
いらいらしていること	136
いらだち	19
イリガトール	67
イリゲーター	6
医療依存	33
医療援助プログラム	50
医療過誤	2
医療観察法	17
医療給付	50
医療計画	50
医療事故	2
医療社会学	57
医療政策	2
医療センター	51
医療ソーシャルワーカー	45, 82
医療保険制度	45
医療補助員	83
衣類	103
入れ歯	66, 103
胃瘻	4
陰影	137
陰茎	120
咽喉	118
インスリン	4, 46
インスリン感受性試験	159
陰性	167
院長	81
咽頭	118
院内学級	11
院内感染	2
インフォームド・コンセント	2
インフルエンザ	152
インフルエンザ治療薬	95

う

ウィメンズヘルス	58
ウイルス性肝炎	153
ウエスト	113
うおのめ	152
うがい薬	95
受付係	83
右心室	118
右心房	118
うずき	143
内の	166
うっ血	138
うっ積	24
うつ病	17
腕	113
膿	140
うろこ状の	140
ウロビリノーゲン	158
浮気	7
上唇	112
上まぶた	112
運動	104
運動失調	136
運動療法	173

え

永久歯	121
エイズ	153
エイズ対策特別計画	54
エイズ予防法	54
衛生学	53
衛生検査官	53
衛生検査所	51
衛生指導員	53
栄養剤	93
栄養士	82
栄養失調〔症〕	5
栄養指導	32
栄養チューブ	6
会陰切開術	26
エストロゲン	26
エネルギー療法	174
エプロン	103
エボラ出血熱	153
襟首	112
エレベーター	63
遠近両用眼鏡	66
園芸療法	173
嚥下障害	5, 39
怨恨	19
円座	68
塩素	160

延命治療		5

お

横隔膜		118
応急処置		171
横行結腸		119
横指		169
黄疸		135
嘔吐		134
嘔吐盆		68
黄斑変性		150
オウム病		153
オーバーベッドテーブル		64
悪寒		134
奥歯		121
臆病		137
お尻洗浄器		64
悪心		134
汚染		53
汚染された		53
おたふく風邪		11
落ちこぼれ		34
落ち着かないこと		136
神経過敏		136
おでき		141
おなかがはること		138
おならをならす		99
オブラート		93
お守り毛布		14
おむつ		38
オムツかぶれ		13
重苦しさ		19
おもちゃ		14
親知らず		121
親の離婚		34
親指		113
おりもの		22
音楽療法士		82
音楽療法		174
音叉		162
温泉療法		173
温熱治療		173
温浴療法		173

か

ガーゼ		65
臥位		175
会計係		83
会計窓口		63
介護機器		46
介護給付		46
介護支援		45
介護保険		45
外耳		120
外耳道		120
外出する		104
回旋		23
階段		63
懐中電灯		69, 103
回腸		119
外転		167, 175
外泊する		104
回復室		63
外来看護		2
外来治療		51
外来窓口		63
カイロプラクティック		174
カウンセラー		33
カウンセリング		3
顔		112
下顎		112
化学療法		5, 173
かかと		114
かかりつけ医		45
過換気		167
可逆性の		142
隔日		92
学習障害		12
額帯鏡		69
喀痰検査		155
拡張期血圧		168
角膜		120
角膜炎		151
隔離		53
かご		64
下行結腸		119
過呼吸		167
火災報知機		62
かさぶた		141
仮死		23
餓死		40
華氏度		167
過食		19
過食症		17
下垂体		122
風邪薬		95
家族看護		2, 57
家族の介護		40

家族の死	40	コー検査	157
家族の病気	7	ガラス棒	162
家族療法	18, 174	カリウム	160
過疎地域医療	32	顆粒剤	94
肩	112	過量	93
下大静脈	118	軽い	142
片言	13	軽い痛み	143
肩こり	136	カルシウム	160
学級閉鎖	33	眼圧測定	158
喀血	137	顔位	23
学校環境衛生	33	簡易更年期指数	26
学校検診	33	肝炎	149, 153
学校保健	57	眼科	84
活性化部分トロンボプラスチン時間	161	眼科医	84
葛藤	19	眼科検査	158
合併症	5	がん看護	2, 38, 57
括約筋	117	肝機能検査	157
かつら	103	眼球	120
家庭医	82	眼球運動	168
家庭医学	83	環境衛生	53
家庭環境	34	緩下剤	95
家庭常備薬	93	間欠自己導尿	11
家庭内暴力	19, 34	間欠熱	167
家庭の崩壊	34	肝硬変	149
家庭の方針	35	看護科学	56
家庭不和	34	看護学概論	56
家庭崩壊	34	看護過程	55
家庭用妊娠検査	21	看護監査委員会	56
カテーテル	162	看護管理	57
カテーテル感染症	5	看護技術	58
カテーテル閉塞	4	看護教育〔学〕	57
カテーテル法	4, 172	看護計画	55
悲しみ	19, 41	看護研究	57
蚊に刺されたあと	135	看護研究法	57
カフ	67	看護実習	58
カプセル	94	看護実習生	82
花粉症	150	看護師免許	52
下方の	166	看護社会学	57
かまれた跡	151	看護情報学	56
我慢できない	142	看護職員需給見通し	52
紙オムツ	66	看護助手	82
かみそり	101	看護診断	55
噛む	99	寛骨	116
カモード	102	看護提供システム	58
粥	99	看護データベース	56
かゆみ	134, 140	看護部長	81
かゆみ止め	96	看護補助員	82
カラードップラー法による心エ		看護面接	55
		看護理論	56

看護倫理	58
鉗子	66
監視装置	68
患者―看護師関係	55
患者―部負担制度	50
患者調査	54
冠状動脈	118
冠状動脈疾患	148
冠状動脈疾患集中治療室	63
間食	100
汗疹	141
関節	117
関節炎	147
関節造影	156
関節痛	136
関節リウマチ	147
関節リウマチ試験	156
汗腺	121
感染管理	2
感染管理看護	57
感染症	32
感染性の	53
完全静脈栄養	4
感染性医療廃棄物	53
感染予防	2
肝臓	119
肝臓がん	149
乾燥した	140
乾燥肌	140
眼帯	65
がん対策	51
浣腸	3, 172
浣腸〔器〕	68
眼痛	139
眼底検査	158
乾皮症	151
カンファレンス	3
漢方薬	93
顔面紅潮	27
顔面神経痛	148
丸薬	94
管理師長	81
緩和	40
緩和ケア	38, 41
緩和療法	173

き

キーパーソン	45
気が遠くなる	136
気管	118
義眼	66
気管支	118
気管支炎	148
気管支拡張薬	95
気管支鏡	162
気管支鏡検査	156
気管支収縮薬	95
気管切開	6
気胸	148
危険物廃棄ボックス	67
気候療法	173
義歯	67
義肢	6
希死念慮	16
義手	66
記述された指示	55
起床時間	103
傷跡	141
傷ついた	140
きずな	13
犠牲者	42
寄生虫	53
――の検査	158
気絶	40, 136
基礎看護〔学〕	56
義足	66
基礎体温	22
貴重品	103
吃音	135
ぎっくり腰	136
気付け薬	93
喫茶室	64
気道確保	12
気道閉塞	12
ギプス	67
ギプス固定	6
気分がゆれていること	136
気分障害	17
気分転換	40
偽薬	93
虐待	19
客観的所見	55
吸引	171
吸引器	67, 68
吸引分娩	24
救急医療	171
救急医療士	83
救急医療システム	52

語	ページ
救急医療隊員	2, 83
救急看護	57
救急救命士	51
救急車	63
救急蘇生	2
救急病棟	62
救護技術	2
臼歯	121
急性期医療	2
急性期看護	57
急性疾患	5
急性の	142
急性リンパ性白血病	12
休息ケア	42
吸痰	38, 46
ギューッという痛み	143
吸入	171
吸入器	67, 94
救命薬	93
救急ワゴン	68
ギュッと握る	13
脅威	18
胸囲	168
教育計画	55
共依存	16
仰臥位	175
強肝薬	95
狂犬病	153
凝固時間	161
胸骨	116
強心剤	96
狭心症	148
胸髄の	169
矯正歯科	84
矯正歯科医	84
胸腺	122
胸帯	65
胸椎	116
胸椎の	169
胸痛	137
恐怖	18
胸部	167
胸部X線検査	155
強膜	120
狂乱	137
局所麻酔	171
局所薬	96
極度の疲労	41
局部的な痛み	143
極量	93
虚弱	134
拒食	19
拒食症	17
巨大児	24
居宅療養管理指導	45
去痰薬	95
拒否	41
切り傷	151
きりきりする痛み	143
筋萎縮性側索硬化症	5
緊急手術	171
緊急避難経路	53
緊急避難所	53
近視	151
近親者の死	40
金属製の物	103
緊張	137
緊張感	136
筋電図検査	156
筋肉	117
──のけいれん	136
筋肉減少症	39
筋肉弛緩薬	96
筋肉注射	171
筋肉痛	136

く

語	ページ
空腸	119
空腹時	93
空腹時血糖	159
空腹時性低血糖	158
くし	101
くしゃみ	137
薬指	113
ぐずる	13
口	112
唇	112
駆虫薬	95
クッシング病	152
靴ずれ	141
首	112
──がすわる	13
首筋	112
くも膜下出血	147
クラッシュカート	68
クランプ	66
グリーフケア	4
クリーム剤	94

クリティカル・パス法	55
グループホーム	37
車椅子	6, 67
クレアチニン	161
グロブリン	160
訓練等給付	46

け

毛穴	121
ケアプラン	46
ケアマネージャー	45
ケアワーカー	45
経過記録	55
計画	55
頸管	26
経管栄養	100
経管栄養剤	3
経管栄養法	3
頸管展退度	26
経口避妊薬	22
経口ブドウ糖負荷試験	159
経口輸液療法	172
脛骨	117
芸術療法	174
軽食	100
頸髄の	169
形成外科	84
形成外科医	84
形成外科手術	172
計測器	162
携帯酸素ボンベ	46
携帯電話	104
携帯用輸液システム	46
傾聴	16, 39
頸椎	116
頸椎の	169
軽度認知障害	39
軽度の	142
経鼻胃管	68
経鼻胃管栄養法	4
軽微な	142
計量カップ	68
計量スプーン	68
けいれん	134, 147
ケースワーカー	45
外科	83
外科医	83
外科的治療	173
外科用メス	66
激痛	141, 143
劇薬	93
化粧	101
化粧水	101
下水処理施設	54
血圧	155, 167
血圧計	67
血液型	159
血液凝固阻止薬	96
血液製剤	51
血液標本	159
血液量	159
結核	148
結核・感染症サーベイランスシステム	53
血管	118
血管拡張薬	96
血管収縮薬	96
血管心臓造影	157
血管性認知症	38
血管造影	157
血球容量	160
月経	21
── がある	21
── がない	21
月経異常	33
月経過多	22
月経困難症	21, 33
月経前症候群	21
結婚	7
── の破たん	7
血色素量	160
決して〜ない	142
血漿	122, 160
血小板	122, 160
血清	160
血清検査	160
血糖検査	159
血尿	139
げっぷ	138
── をする	99
血便	138
結膜	120
結膜炎	150
血友病	152
解毒	171
解毒剤	96
ケトン体	158
解熱薬	95

下痢	5, 138, 149
ケリーパッド	65
下痢止め薬	95
腱	117
検疫	53
減塩食	100
幻覚	136
検眼鏡	162
献血	51
肩甲骨	116
健康寿命	37
健康障害	38
健康診断	33
健康増進	52
健康増進法	52
健康保険	50
健康保険証	104
言語療法	173
言語療法士	82
検査室	63
検死	42
犬歯	121
原始反射	11
研修医	82
現症	166
腱鞘炎	147
健診	13
検体立て	68
幻聴	136
腱反射	156
顕微鏡	162
検便	157

こ

恋人との別れ	6
コインランドリー	62
抗アレルギー薬	96
更衣	104
抗うつ剤	17
公害	53
口蓋垂	118
口蓋裂	12
光覚	168
睾丸	120
抗がん剤	96
交感神経	117
後期高齢者医療制度	37, 45
口腔ケア	6
高血圧	138

抗血液凝固薬	96
高血糖	5
膠原病	152
抗高血圧薬	95
虹彩	120
口臭	141
公衆衛生	32, 53
公衆衛生審議会	51
公衆衛生法	54
甲状腺	122
甲状腺刺激ホルモン	158
口唇が乾いていること	135
抗真菌薬	95
向神経薬	17
口唇裂	12
向精神薬	17
厚生年金	50
抗生物質	95
厚生労働省	51
光線療法	173
交代性無呼吸	137
高タンパク食	100
紅潮した	140
硬直	134, 135
交通事故	7
公的資金	50
後天性の	7
喉頭	118
喉頭蓋	118
行動療法	174
口内炎	141
高熱	167
更年期	26
更年期障害	26
抗ヒスタミン薬	96
抗貧血薬	96
項部透過像	22
興奮	19, 137
硬膜外ブロック	24
肛門	119
膏薬	94
抗利尿ホルモン	159
抗利尿薬	95
高齢化社会	37
高齢者総合機能評価	37
高齢者肺炎	39
高齢出産	23
誤嚥	39
氷枕	66

股間	113
呼吸	168
呼吸音	169
呼吸管理	46
呼吸器科	83
呼吸器専門医	83
呼吸窮迫症候群	11
呼吸困難	137
呼吸数	134, 168
国際看護師協会	56
黒色腫	151
国民皆保険制度	50
国民健康保険	45
国立病院	51
国立病院機構	51
固形食	100
心のケア	16, 39
心の健康	16
心の闇	18
個室	62
五十肩	147
個人療法	174
姑息的手術	172
子育て支援	24
誇大妄想	19
骨髄	122
骨髄バンク	51
骨折	147
骨粗鬆症	39, 147
骨盤	26, 116
骨盤位	23
コップ	162
〜ごと	92
孤独	18
孤独感	40
子どもの死	7
子どもの独立	7
粉薬・散剤	94
こぶ	141, 151
鼓膜	120
小枕	67
ゴミ箱	64, 104
ゴミ袋	104
ゴム製手袋	65
米	99
こめかみ	112
小指	113
こり	134
コルセット	67
コルチゾン・ブドウ糖負荷試験	159
コレステロール降下薬	96
コレラ	152
婚姻率	54
根拠に基づく医療	56
根拠に基づく看護	56
昏睡	137
コンタクトレンズ	103
根治手術	172
根治療法	174
混乱	134

さ

坐位	175
災害	53
災害看護	2
災害救助法	53
災害対策	53
細菌検査	156
最近親者	40
採血室	63
採血用ホルダー	67
サイコロジカルファーストエイド	18
再婚	7
菜食主義者	100
再生医療	173
砕石位	175
臍帯	24
在宅介護支援センター	46
在宅看護	57
在宅緩和医療	45
在宅ケア	46
在宅酸素療法	46
在宅人工呼吸法	46
在宅中心静脈栄養	46
在宅福祉対策	45
在宅モニタリングシステム	46
在宅療養指導管理料	46
サイトメガロウイルス感染症	26
催乳反射	25
採尿器	68
細胞検査	156
催眠療法	173
作業療法	173
作業療法士	82
搾乳器	24
鎖骨	116
坐骨神経	117

刺し傷	151		色覚検査	158
さしこみ	143		磁気共鳴画像法	155
差込プラグ	68		色彩療法	174
差込み便器	67		子宮	26, 120
差し込むような痛み	143		子宮外妊娠	25
挫傷	151		子宮がん	25
左心室	118		子宮筋腫	25
左心房	118		子宮頸がん	25
嗄声	137		子宮出血	25
擦過創	151		子宮内胎児発育遅延	25
殺菌剤	65		子宮内膜掻爬術	26
殺人	40		子宮復古	24
里親	35		事業の開始	7
寒け	134		しくしくする痛み	143
坐薬	3, 94		止血	171
皿	100		止血帯	67
ザラザラした	140		試験管	66
サルコペニア	39		歯垢	141
産科	84		耳甲介	120
産科医	84		自己決定権	3
三角巾	67		自己嫌悪	41
産科ショック	23		死後硬直	42
産業保健	2		事故死	40
産後うつ	26		自己尊重	39
三叉神経	117		自己注射	46
産褥期	23		自己導尿	4
酸素タンク	68		自己否定	41
酸素プラグ差込口	64		しこり	27
酸素マスク	66		自殺	16, 40
産道	23		自殺願望	16
散瞳	151		自殺企図	16
散髪	101		死産	23
散発性の	142		思春期	33
サンプル	54		思春期早発症	33
			思春期遅発症	33
し			思春期妊娠	33
自意識過剰	19		自傷	16
シーツ	64, 103		死傷者	42
歯科	84		視診	166
歯科医	84		視神経	117
耳介	120		指数弁	169
歯科衛生士	82		歯石	152
歯科技工士	83		指節骨	116
視覚のぼけ	140		自然死	40
子癇	26		事前指示〔書〕	40
歯冠	67		死前喘鳴	41
耳管	121		歯槽膿漏症	152
子癇前症	25		持続性の	142
時間治療	174		自尊心	19, 39

舌	119	自分でないような状態	135
下着	103	自閉症	18
下唇	112	死への準備教育	
下まぶた	112	脂肪酸	161
市町村保健センター	51	死亡証明書	41
弛張熱	167	死亡診断書	41
歯痛	141	死亡率	27
刺痛	143	しみ	141
耳痛	139	事務職員	83
膝蓋腱反射	169	シムズ体位	175
膝蓋骨	117	事務長	81
失業	6	視野	168
膝胸位	175	シャーレ	66
失禁	38, 139	斜位の	166
湿気のある	140	社会的孤立	19
失語	136	社会福祉	52
実施	55	社会福祉士	2
湿潤な	140	社会復帰	46
失神	136	社会保険の福祉施設	52
湿疹	141	弱視	150
質の管理	55	蛇口	102
湿布	172	視野検査	158
疾病関連群	55	斜視	151
疾病予防	32	借金	6
失明	151	しゃっくりをする	99
失恋	6	尺骨	116
児童虐待	34	シャワーキャップ	101
児童憲章	35	シャワー室	62
児童相談所	35	シャワー浴介助	102
自動体外式除細動器	6	集学的治療	6
自動販売機	62	充血	24
児童福祉	35	充血した目	139
児童扶養手当	35	周産期	23
児童養護施設	35	周産期死亡率	54
死と臨終	41	周産期センター	63
歯肉	168	収縮期血圧	167
死にゆく過程の5段階	41	重症急性呼吸器症候群	153
視能訓練士	82	就職	7
死の本能	41	就職難	34
死の看取り	41	就寝の準備	103
死のもがき	41	住宅購入	7
しばしば	142	住宅ローン	6
死斑	42	集団感染	33
市販薬	93	集団検診	32
耳鼻咽喉科	84	集団療法	174
耳鼻咽喉科医	84	集中治療看護	57
慈悲殺	40	集中治療室	63
しびれ感	136	重篤な	142
しびん	68	十二指腸	119

十二指腸潰瘍	149	錠剤	94
就眠時	93	硝子体	120
絨毛膜下血腫	25	上司とのトラブル	6
主観的幸福感を見る尺度	155	症状	166
主観的所見	55	──の発現	135
縮瞳	151	昇進	7
受験の失敗	34	上大静脈	118
手根骨	116	使用中	102
授産施設	17	小腸	119
主治医	82	消灯時間	103
手術	171	床頭台	64
手術看護	57	消毒液	65
手術室	62	消毒剤	65, 96
手術室看護	57	消毒綿	65
手術専門看護師	81	消毒用アルコール	96
手術台	68	小児科	84
手術用着衣	65	小児科医	84
受精卵	21	小児がん	12
受胎調節	22	小児看護〔学〕	56
出血	135	小児気管支喘息	12
出血時間	161	小児麻痺	11
術後食	100	小脳	117
出産	7	情報システム	54
出生前検査	23	上方の	166
出生率	27	静脈	168
出席停止	35	静脈注射	171
手動弁	169	蒸留水	65
授乳	24	上腕	113
主任看護師	81	上腕骨	116
受容	41	ショートステイ	37
腫瘍摘出手術	172	職業保健	57
手浴	101	食後	92
潤滑剤表面麻酔剤	4	食事介助	100
循環器科	83	食事時間	99
循環器専門医	83	食事中	93
准看護師	81	食事の指針	35
消炎薬	95	食事のセッティング	100
障害	5	食事療法	6, 173
障害基礎年金	52	触診	166
障害者自立支援法	16	食前	92
障害者地域生活支援センター	17	褥瘡	141
消火器	62	食中毒	5, 149
消化器科	83	食堂	64
消化器専門医	83	食道	119
消化剤	95	食道鏡検査	157
松果腺	122	食品衛生	53
蒸気吸入器	68	食品管理	32
症候群	166	食品取扱業者	53
上行結腸	119	食物アレルギー	11

食欲減退	138	人口呼吸装置	68
食欲亢進	135	人工受精	21
食欲不振	19, 135	人工装具	66
除細動器	67	人口調査	54
助産学	56	人口動態統計	54
助産師	22, 82	人工妊娠中絶	22
処置室	62	心呼吸系	167
処置台	68	心雑音	168
処置用具	67	診察券	104
食間	92	診察室	62
初乳	25	心身症	18
処方箋	93	心身障害者福祉協会	52
徐脈	138, 167	新生児	10
自立支援	11, 16	新生児期	24
試料	54	新生児行動評価	10
視力	168	新生児室	63
視力検査	34, 158	新生児集中治療室	10
視力検査表	162	新生児蘇生	13
耳漏	139	新生児低血糖	12
シロップ剤	94	心尖	118
白っぽい	140	振せん	137
しわ	141	心臓	118
心因性の	16	── のバイパス手術	172
腎盂炎	150	腎臓	119
腎炎	149	心臓カテーテル検査	157
心音	168	心臓死	40
心音図検査	157	心臓手術	172
新患受付	63	心臓病	148
腎機能検査	158	心臓病食	100
鍼灸治療	174	腎臓病食	100
心筋炎	148	心臓ペースメーカー	174
心筋梗塞	148	心臓発作	148
心筋症	148	親族	40
寝具	103	靭帯	117
寝具一式	64	身体検査	155
真空採血管	67	身体障害者	52
神経	117, 169	診断計画	55
神経科	84	身長	168
神経科医	84	身長計	34, 69
神経症	18	陣痛	23
神経衰弱	17	心的外傷後ストレス障害	18
神経性食欲不振症	17	心的外傷体験	19
神経痛	148	心電図	157
人口	54	心肺蘇生	13
人工栄養	14	心拍数	168
人工器官	66	真皮	121
人工喉頭	6	深部腱反射	169
人工呼吸	171	心不全	148
人工呼吸器	68	腎不全	150

じんましん	141, 152
診療所	32, 51
心理療法	173

す

膵炎	149
衰弱	34, 136
水晶体	120
膵臓	119
水痘	11
水道施設	54
水頭症	12
水分	100
水分補給	100
水泡音	137
髄膜	117
睡眠パターンの調整	103
睡眠薬	17
ずきずきする痛み	143
スクールカウンセリング	33
スクリーニング検査	155
頭痛	134
ステロイド	11, 96
ストーマ	4
ストレス	18
ストレス性失禁	139
ストレステスト	156
ストレッチャー	67
すね	114
スプーン1杯	93
スプレー剤	94
すり傷	151
スリッパ	103
すりむいた	140

せ

生育支援	10
生化学血液検査	160
生活訓練施設	17
生活の質	55
正看護師	81
性感染症	34, 153
正期産	23
性器出血	25
性教育	33
整形外科	83
整形外科医	83
生検	155
性交	21
性交痛	21
制酸剤	95
清拭	101
生児出生	10
正常出産	23
生殖器	114
精神安定剤	17
精神科	84
精神科医	84
精神科薬物療法	18
精神科リエゾン看護	57
精神看護〔学〕	56
成人看護〔学〕	56
精神疾患	17
精神障害者	16
精神遅滞	11
精神保健センター	51
精神保健福祉士	2
精神保健福祉法	16
ぜいぜい息をすること	137
性腺機能低下症	12
性腺刺激ホルモン	159
声帯	118
生体移植手術	172
正中	169
成長曲線	34
整腸剤	95
成長障害	12, 34
成長ホルモン	33, 158
成長ホルモン治療	12
性的不能	3
性と生殖にかかわる健康	21
制吐薬	95
成年後見制度	17
整髪	101
生命維持装置の停止	42
生命表	54
性欲	3
性欲減退	3
生理学的機能検査	155
生理機能検査室	63
生理食塩液	94
生理痛	22
生理不順	22
生理用ナプキン	22
世界保健機関	50
セカンドオピニオン	3
赤外線療法	173
脊髄	117

脊髄造影	156
脊椎	116
咳止めシロップ	95
咳止め薬	95
舌圧子	66
切開	172
舌下製剤	94
赤血球	122, 160
赤血球数	160
赤血球沈降速度	160
石鹸	101
切歯	121
摂氏度	167
摂食準備	100
摂食障害	17
切石位	175
切迫流産	25
絶望	41, 137
背中	113
——の痛み	136
背骨	116
セルフケア	46
洗顔	101
洗顔クリーム	101
前駆期	16
全血球計算値	160
潜血試験	158
仙骨	116
仙骨の	169
洗剤	102
洗浄器	67
染色体異常	25
先進医療	3
全身状態	166
全人的苦痛	4
全身の痛み	143
全身麻酔	171
仙髄の	169
喘息	148
喘息治療薬	95
洗濯室	62
洗濯物	102
洗濯物袋	102
前置胎盤	24
疝痛	11, 143
先天性股関節脱臼	12
先天性食道閉鎖症	12
先天性の	7
前頭側頭型認知症	38

洗髪	101
洗髪車	68
洗面器	101
洗面所	62
洗面用具	101
せん妄	5, 137
泉門	13
専門看護師	81
専門職種間連携	45
前立腺	120
前立腺がん	150
前腕	113

そ

瘡	140
総入れ歯	66
躁うつ病	17
造影剤	162
挿管	172
臓器移植	3, 172
臓器移植法	52
臓器提供	52
雑巾	104
装具	66
装具装着	6
造血薬	96
総合受付	63
総合診療	32
総合病院	51
総コレステロール	161
早産	23
葬式の準備	42
喪失	135
喪失感	41
躁状態	19
総蛋白	160
蒼白な	140
躁病	17
総ビリルビン	161
相補療法	173
掻痒感	11
疎外感	18
側臥位	175
続発症	5
側方の	166
速脈	167
足浴	101
足浴用洗面器	69
鼠径部	113

蘇生処置を拒絶すること	41
卒業	35
足根骨	117
外の	166
そばかす	141
尊厳	39
尊厳死	40
存在価値	39

た

ターナー症候群	12
ターミナルケア	37
第2次性徴	33
体位交換	38
体位変換器	6
退院支援	4, 32
退院指導	4
ダイオキシン	53
体温	155, 167
体温計	68
胎芽	26
体外受精	21
代替医療	173
代替医療プラクティショナー	51
体格指数	4, 34
大気質指数	54
退行	19
胎児	10
――の発達	10
胎児仮死	10, 23
胎児心拍	10
胎児治療	26
体脂肪率	34
胎児モニタリング	10
体臭	141, 168
体重	168
体重計	34, 69
体重増加	10
大静脈造影	157
対症療法	172
退職	7
対耳輪	120
対人関係療法	18
対人恐怖	19
大腿骨	116
大腿部	114
大腸	119
大腸炎	149
大腸がん	149
大腸鏡検査	157
大動脈	118
大動脈造影	157
大動脈瘤	149
大脳	117
胎盤	26, 120
胎盤早期剥離	25
体表面積	168
胎便	24
大便	102
ダウン症候群	12
耐えうる	142
耐え難い	142
唾液	119, 141
タオル	101
抱きしめる	13
タクシー乗り場	64
宅配サービス	46
打診	166
多胎妊娠	25
脱臼	147
脱脂綿	65
脱水	13
脱水症	5
脱水症状	134
脱腸帯	68
タッチ療法	174
脱毛	3
脱毛症	151
脱力感	135
多尿	139, 150
多発性の	7
打撲傷	151
打撲症	151
魂	40
痰	137
担架	67
胆管結石	149
たんこぶ	151
胆汁尿〔症〕	150
胆石〔症〕	149
断続的な	142
痰壺	68
胆の	119
胆のう炎	149
蛋白結合ヨウ素	159
蛋白尿〔症〕	150
タンポン	22, 65
談話室	62

ち

チアノーゼ	3, 134
地域医療連携システム	32
地域看護学	56
地域包括ケア	32
地域保健医療計画	51
チーム医療	33
チェーンストークス呼吸	137
ちくちく刺すような痛み	143
蓄尿器	68
乳首	113
智歯	121
致死量	93
腟	26, 120
腟炎	25
窒息死	40
腟内診	22
血の塊	5
着床	21
注意欠陥過活動性障害	12
中核症状	39
中耳	120
中耳炎	150
注射器	6, 66
注射針	6, 66
中手骨	116
昼食	99
中心静脈栄養法	4
虫垂	119
虫垂炎	149
中性脂肪	161
中足骨	117
中程度の	142
中毒	134
中毒事故管理センター	54
注入器	67
腸炎	149
超音波	22
超音波検査	155
徴候	166
超高齢社会	37
腸雑音	169
朝食	99
聴診	166
聴診器	68, 162
調節	166
超低出生体重児	10
腸捻転	149
腸閉塞	149
調味料	100
聴力計	162
聴力検査	34, 158
直接型ビリルビン	161
直腸	119
直腸がん	149
直腸鏡	162
直腸診	23
ちょっとした痛み	143
治療計画	55
治療食	100
治療優先順位の選別	51
鎮静	39
鎮静剤	17
鎮痛剤	42, 95

つ

痛風	152
杖	67
疲れやすいこと	135
突き指	136
常に	142
ツベルクリン反応	11
つまようじ	100
爪痕	151
爪切り	101
吊り包帯	66
つわり	23

て

手	113
——の甲	113
——のひら	113
低栄養	39
帝王切開	24
低換気	167
デイケア	37
低血圧	138
低血糖	5
デイサービス	37
低酸素血症	168
低出生体重	10
ティッシュペーパー	102
剃毛	172
適格性	50
摘出手術	172
摘便	172
手首	113

デス・エデュケーション	41
鉄	161
手に負えない	142
てんかん	5, 148
点眼薬	94
電気器具	104
電気ショック療法	174
電気毛布	64
デング熱	153
転校	35
点字器	6
電子顕微鏡	162
伝染病	5
伝染病対策	53
伝染病棟	62
伝染病予防法	54
転地療法	174
点滴	171
点滴用ポール	67
転倒防止	38
転倒リスク評価	38
点鼻薬	94
殿部	113
電話指示	55

と

トイレ	62, 102
トイレットペーパー	102
トイレトレーニング	11
頭囲	168
同意書	104
頭蓋	116
動悸	137
瞳孔	120
瞳孔散大	140, 151
統合失調症	17
瞳孔反射	158
瞳孔不同	166
橈骨	116
透析	172
疼痛管理	3
疼痛処理	42
糖尿	139
糖尿病	152
糖尿病食	100
頭髪	112
頭部	112
動物介在療法	174
動脈	168

投薬量	93
動揺	137
トータルペイン	4
時折起こる	142
ときどき	142
ときどき起こる	142
特定看護師	81
特別食	99
特別養護老人ホーム	37
吐血	138
床ずれ	40, 141
特効薬	93
突然死	40
ドップラー超音波検査	157
ドメスティックバイオレンス	34
共にいること	39
どもり	135
吐薬	95
ドライアイ	139
ドライヤー	102
トラコーマ	150
トリアージ	3
鳥インフルエンザ	153
トリグリセリド	161
鳥肌	141
取り引き	41
トレイ	68, 100
トレッドミル試験	157
トレンデレンブルグ体位	175
トローチ剤	94
トロンビン時間	161
トロンボテスト	161
トロンボプラスチン抑制試験	161
鈍痛	143

な

ナースコール	64
ナースステーション	62
内科	83
内科医	83
内科的治療	173
内耳	121
内視鏡	66, 162
内視鏡検査	157
内視鏡検査室	63
内視鏡手術	172
内診	22
内転	167, 175
内分泌科	83

内分泌専門医	83	妊娠中毒症	25
治りにくい	142	妊娠糖尿病	25
中指	113	認知機能低下	38
亡くなる	40	認知行動療法	18
ナチュラルキラー細胞	122	認知症	18, 38
ナトリウム	160	——の中核症状と心理症状	39
涙目	139	認知療法	173
軟膏	94	妊婦	21
難聴	139	妊婦健診	21
なんとか我慢できる	142		
難病	5		

ぬ・ね

		ぬるま湯	65
		寝汗	135

に

		ネグレクト	19
にきび	140	寝言をいう	99
憎しみ	19	寝小便	11
西ナイル熱	153	寝たきり老人	38
二重視	151	寝たきり老人ゼロ作戦	38
日光浴	104	熱	134
二頭筋反射	169	熱傷	151
日本医師会	52	熱性けいれん	11
日本看護協会	56	熱湯	65
日本赤十字社	52	ネフローゼ	150
入院受付	63	練り歯磨き	101
入学	35	粘液	137
乳がん	26	粘液分泌過多	137
乳歯	121	ねんざ	147
——が生えること	13	ねんねタオル	14
乳児死亡率	27	ノイローゼ	18
乳汁分泌	24		
乳児用ミルク	14		

の

乳腺炎	26		
乳房	113	脳	117
入眠介助	103	脳幹	117
乳幼児突然死症候群	12	脳外科手術	172
入浴	101	脳血栓症	147
入浴介助	102	脳梗塞	147
尿	102	脳死	3, 40
尿意促迫	139	脳腫瘍	12, 148
尿管	119	脳神経	169
尿検査	158	脳神経外科	83
尿酸	161	脳神経外科医	83
尿素窒素	160	脳しんとう〔症〕	148
尿道	119	脳性麻痺	25
尿量過少	150	脳脊髄液検査	156
尿路感染症	150	脳卒中	147
尿路結石	150	脳〔内〕出血	147
妊娠	7, 21	膿尿	150
妊娠検査	21	膿尿症	150
妊娠高血圧症候群	25	脳波検査	156

脳貧血	148
のけ者	34
喉の痛み	134
喉の乾き	135
のどぼとけ	112
伸びる	99
のぼせ	135
飲み込む	99
ノロウイルス	153

は

歯	121
パーキンソン病	5, 39
肺	118
胚	26
肺炎	148
背横位	175
徘徊	38
背臥位	175
肺活量計	162
肺活量測定検査	156
肺がん	148
肺気腫	148
肺機能検査	156
配偶者の死	40
排水チューブ	67
排泄介助	102
バイタルサイン	3
売店	64
梅毒	153
排尿	102
排尿困難	139, 150
排尿障害	150
はいはい歩きする	13
排便	102
排便反射	11
敗北感	41
廃用症候群	39
排卵	21
排卵誘発剤	21
ハイリスク児	10
排臨	24
パウダー剤	94
はかり	69
吐き気	134
歯茎	121
白内障	150
はげ〔頭〕	141
激しい	142

激しい痛み	142
激しい腹痛	11
箱庭療法	173
破産	7
はし	100
はしか	11
橋本甲状腺炎	152
パジャマ	103
播種性血管内凝固症候群	25
破水	23
バスタオル	101
バスローブ	64
バセドー氏病	152
肌荒れ	140
蜂刺され	135
白血球	122, 160
白血病	12, 152
発生率	54
発達看護	10
発達障害	17
鼻	112
──をかむ	99
鼻血	139
鼻詰まり	139
鼻水	134, 139
花屋	64
パニック	19
パパニコローテスト	22
歯ブラシ	101
歯磨き	101
腹	113
腹帯	65
バラ疹	141
バリウム注腸	157
パルスオキシメーター	6, 46
腫れ	135
パン	100
半月	113
番号	166
反射	169
絆創膏	65
半側麻痺	148
バンドエイド	65
半ファウラー体位	175
反復流産	25
半分	93

ひ

冷え	134

鼻炎	150
被害妄想	19
日帰り手術	172
皮下組織	121
皮下注射	171
光過敏症	140, 148
光恐怖〔症〕	148
引きこもり	16
ひきつけ	134
鼻腔	121
ひげそりクリーム	101
ひげを剃ること	101
鼻孔	112
腓骨	117
尾骨	116
膝	114
肘	113
皮脂腺	121
比重	158
非常口	62
非常用ベル	102
皮疹	140
非侵襲的陽圧換気	4
ヒスタミン薬	96
ヒステリー症	18
脾臓	122
額	112
ビタミンK欠乏症	26
ビタミン剤	93
左の	166
悲嘆	41
悲嘆回復	4
悲嘆ケア	39
鼻中隔	121
鼻痛	139
引越し	7
必要に応じて	92
ひどい痛み	142
ヒトゲノムプロジェクト	51
人差し指	113
ヒト絨毛性ゴナドトロピン	159
皮内注射	171
泌尿器科	84
泌尿器科医	84
避妊	22
否認	41
避妊具	22
避妊ペッサリー	22
避妊薬	22

避妊リング	22
微熱	167
ひび	152
ひび割れた	140
皮膚科	84
皮膚科医	84
皮膚がん	151
肥満	135
冷や汗	135
百日咳	11
病衣	64
評価	55
病室	62
美容整形	172
病態栄養	3
病的状態	54
病棟師長	81
氷嚢	66
表皮	121
標本	54
病理検査	156
ひりひりすること	134
ピル	22
昼寝	103
疲労感	135
貧血	24, 152
ピンセット	66
頻尿	139
頻拍	138
頻脈	138, 167
ひんやりしている	140

ふ

ファイバー気管支鏡検査	156
ファイバースコープ	162
ファイバー内視鏡検査	158
ファウラー体位	175
不安	18, 136
不安障害	17
不安神経症	18
フィジカルアセスメント	3
フィブリノーゲン	161
フィブリン分解産物	161
風疹	11
不快	19
不可逆性の	142
不感症	3
不機嫌	135
腹囲	168

副院長	81
腹臥位	175
復学	33
副交感神経	117
副甲状腺	122
副作用	93
福祉	37
複視	151
福祉国家	52
福祉人材バンク	52
副腎	122
副腎皮質刺激ホルモン	159
腹痛	138
腹部膨満	5
副木	67
腹膜炎	149
腹膜透析法	4
服薬管理	4
ふくらはぎ	114
ふけ	141
不治の病	40
浮腫	135
不信	41
婦人科	84
婦人科医	84
不整脈	138, 149, 167
豚インフルエンザ	153
普通食	99
二日酔い	135
腹腔鏡	162
腹腔鏡検査	157
フットレール	64
不登校	33
ブドウ糖	160
ブドウ糖負荷試験	159
ふとん	64
不妊症	25
部分トロンボプラスチン時間	161
不眠	19
不眠症	18
不明瞭な話し方をすること	135
プライバシーの保護	4
プライマリーケア	2, 51
プライマリーケア・ナーシング	57
プライマリーナーシング	55
プライマリーナース	81
ブラインド	64
ブラジャー	103
フラストレーション	136
プラセボ	93
震え	137
ふるえ	13, 134
プレイルーム	62
プレドニゾロン・ブドウ糖負荷試験	159
プロゲステロン	26
プロトロンビン時間	161
風呂場	62
プロラクチン	159
分泌物	135
分娩	23
分娩室	23, 63
分娩台	23
分娩予定日	23
噴霧器	68

へ

ヘアブラシ	101
平均血圧	168
平均寿命	54
平均値	54
閉経期	26
へそ	113
――の緒	24
別居	7
ベッド柵	64
ベッドレール	64
ペトリ皿	66
ペニス勃起不能	3
ヘマトクリット値	160
ヘモグロビン	160
ヘルスアセスメント	3
ヘルニアバンド	68
ヘルパー	45
ヘルペス	153
弁	118
便器	102
娩出力	23
偏頭痛	136
扁桃炎	150
扁桃腺	118
便秘	5, 138
片麻痺	148

ほ

保育器	13
縫合	172
膀胱	119

膀胱炎	149	発疹	141
方向感覚を失うこと	136	ホットライン	46
包交車	68	ほてり	135
放射線科	63, 83	──のある	140
放射線科医	83	母乳	14
放射線用プロテクター	162	母乳栄養	14
放射線療法	5, 172	哺乳瓶	14, 24
疱疹	153	──の乳首	14
放心〔状態〕	136	骨	116
防水シート	65	骨と関節	169
包帯	65	ホメオパシー	174
包帯交換ワゴン	68	ボランティア	83
乏尿	139, 150	ポリープ	135
防腐剤	96	ポリオ	11
訪問栄養食事指導	45	ホルター心電計	162
訪問介護	45	ホルモン補充療法	26
訪問看護	32, 57	ホルモン薬	96
訪問看護師	82	ホルモン療法	173
訪問看護ステーション	32, 46		
ほお	112	**ま**	
ポータブルトイレ	68		
ホームヘルパー	45	毎週	92
保温器	13	毎日	92
ぽかぽかしている	140	前歯	121
ほくろ	141	マグネシウム	160
保健機能食品	3	枕	103
保険給付	50	麻酔	171
保健師	32, 53	麻酔科	84
保健師助産師看護師法	52	麻酔科医	84
保健室	33	麻酔看護	57
保健指導	33	麻酔薬	96
保健所	32, 51, 53	マタニティーブルー	22
保健統計学	2	待合室	63
保健福祉政策	58	末期	38, 40
歩行器	6, 67	睫毛	112
母子看護	57	マッサージ療法	173
母子感染	22	末梢神経	117
保湿剤	11	マットレス	64
母子手帳	24	松葉杖	67
ポジトロンCT	155	まばたきする	99
母子の健康	24	麻痺	136
母子保健	24	瞼	112
母子寮	35	眉	112
ホスピス	40	マラリア	152
母性看護	57	慢性疾患	5
母体管理	24	慢性の	142
ボタン	103		
補聴器	66	**み**	
発作	10, 134, 135	味覚芽	119

右の	166
未熟児	13
水	94
水薬	94
水差し	69
水ぶくれ	140
水虫	151
看取り	38
身分証明書	104
見舞い人	104
耳	112
耳あか	139
耳たぶ	112
耳鳴り	139
脈圧	168
脈拍	134, 167
味蕾	119
民生委員	51

む

無意味さ	41
無塩食	100
無関心	41
無気力	41
無月経	21, 33
無呼吸	167
無酸素症	167
虫歯	152
無職	7
むち打ち症	147
無糖食	100
無尿	139, 150
胸	113
——の圧迫感	137
胸当て	14
胸やけ	138
無力感	137

め

目	112
——のかゆみ	140
メガネ	103
目がヒリヒリすること	140
メジャー	68
メタボリックシンドローム	3
めったに～ない	142
めまい	134, 137
目やに	140
メラニン阻害薬	96

メラノーマ	151
免疫〔学的〕検査	156
免疫無防備状態	152
免疫抑制剤	96
免疫療法	173
面会	4
面会時間	104
綿球	65
メンタルヘルス	3
綿棒	65

も

毛球	121
毛根	121
毛細血管	118
盲腸	119
盲腸炎	149
毛布	103
網膜	120
網膜症	150
網膜障害	150
燃え尽き症候群	41
沐浴	24
ものもらい	151
もの忘れ	16
物忘れ	136
問題解決型教育法	56
問題志向型記録の形式	55

や

夜間勤務の看護師	81
夜間多尿〔症〕	150
薬剤師	82
薬草療法	174
薬物依存	19
薬物治療	173
薬物乱用	17
やけど	151
やけど跡	141
焼けるような痛み	143
薬価基準	50
薬局	63, 93
やわらかい	140
軟らかい食事	100

ゆ

憂うつ	17
遊戯療法	174
有効量	93

夕食	99
優生保護法	24
遊離脂肪酸	161
輸血	3, 171
湯たんぽ	66
指関節	113
指サック	65
指しゃぶり	13
指の爪	113
夢をみる	99
ゆるい便通	138

よ

溶液	94
要介護	38
容器	162
養護学校	11
養護教諭	11
養護施設	32
幼児	13
羊水	26, 120
羊水穿刺	22
腰髄の	169
陽性	167
腰椎	116
腰椎の	169
腰痛	136
陽電子放出断層撮影	155
ヨードチンキ	96
抑うつ	17, 41
浴槽	102
よだれをたらす	13, 99
欲求不満	136
予防医学	2
予防接種	33
予防接種法	53
予防注射	13
予防薬	93
嫁姑問題	35
与薬カート	68

ら

ラ音	137
ラテックス手袋	65
卵管	26
乱視	150
ランセット	66
卵巣	120

り

リウマチ	147
リエゾン看護	57
理学療法	173
理学療法士	82
罹患率	54
離婚	7
離婚率	54
リストラ	6
立位	175
離乳食	14, 25
利尿薬	95
理髪店	64
リハビリテーションセンター	63
罹病率	54
リビング・ウィル	4
リフレクソロジー	174
流産	23
流動食	100
留年	34
療育	10
良性の	7
緑内障	150
リラクゼーション	4
リン脂質	161
臨床看護	58
臨床検査技師	82
臨床工学技士	2
臨床心理士	2, 82
リンパ	122
リンパ球	122
リンパ節	122, 169
リンパ腺	122
淋病	153

る・れ

涙管	120
るいそう	135
霊安室	64
冷蔵庫	64
霊的安寧	42
レーザー手術	172
レクリエーション療法	174
レスパイトケア	46
レッグレスト	67
裂傷	151
レビー小体型認知症	38

ろ

廊下	63
老化度	38
老人看護〔学〕	56
老人クラブ	37
老人性痴呆疾患センター	37
老人性認知症	38
老人ホーム	32
老人保健施設	37
老人保健法	37
老年期うつ尺度	38
老年症候群	39
濾過器	69
ロコモティブシンドローム	46
濾紙	65
ロッカー	64
肋間の	169
肋骨	116
ロビー	63

わ

わきが	151
わき毛	113
わきの下	113
わき腹	113
ワクチン	93
ワゴン	100
わずかな	142
わずかに	167
笑い療法	174
椀	100

A

a deep emotional scar	18
a half	93
abdomen	113
abdominal binder	65
abdominal bloating	5
abdominal circumference	168
abdominal pain	138
abduction	167, 175
abnormal bowel sounds	138
abraded wound	151
abrasion	151
abruption placentae	25
absence of menstruation	21, 33
absent-mindedness	136
absorbent cotton	65
abuse	19
acceptance	41
accessory	103
accidental death	40
accommodation	166
acetone	158
ache	134
Achilles' tendon	117
Achilles' tendon reflex	169
acne	140
acquired	7
acquired immunodeficiency syndrome	153
Act on Public Health Nurses, Midwives and Nurses	52
activated partial thromboplastin time	161
acupuncture and moxibustion therapy	174
acute	142
acute disease	5
acute lymphocytic leukemia	12
acute medical care	2
acute-care nursing	57
Adam's apple	112
adduction	167, 175
adhesive bandage	65
adhesive tape	65
adjustment of sleep pattern	103
admission office	63
adolescent pregnancy	33
adrenal gland	122
adrenocorticotropic hormone	159
adult children	16
adult guardianship	17
adult nursing	56
advance directive	40
advanced life support	171
advanced medical care	3
after meals	92
afterbirth	23
aging society	37
agitation	137
agony	41
AIDS Prevention Law	54
air quality index	54
airway management	12
airway obstruction	12
albumin	160

Index

albumin-globulin ratio	160
albuminuria	150
alcohol dependence	19
alcoholism	17
aldosterone	159
alienation	18
allergen elimination	12
allergic reaction	3
allergy	93
alleviation	40
alopecia	151
alternative healthcare practitioner	51
alternative medicine	173
always	142
Alzheimer's disease	38
amblyopia	150
ambulance	63
amenorrhea	21
ammonia	160
amniocentesis	22
amniorrhexis	23
amniotic fluid	26, 120
amyotrophic lateral sclerosis	5
analeptic	93
anemia	24, 152
anesthesia	171
anesthesia nursing	57
anesthesiologist	84
anesthesiology	84
anesthetic	96
anger	19, 41
angina pectoris	148
angiocardiography	157
angiography	157
animal therapy	174
anisocoria	166
ankle	114
ankle jerk	169
anorexia	17, 19, 135
anoxia	167
ante cibos	92
ante cibum	92
antenatal testing	23
anthelmintic	95
anti-flu medicine	95
antiacid	95
antiallergic agent	96
antianemic agent	96
antiasthmatic	95
antibiotic	95
anticoagulant	96
antidepressant	17
antidiarrhetic	95
antidiuretic	95
antidiuretic hormone	159
antidote	96
antiemetic	95
antiflatulent	95
antihelix	120
antihistamines	96
antihypertensive	95
antimycotic agent	95
antiphlogistic	95
antipruritic	96
antipyretic	95
antiseptic	96
antiseptic solution	65
anuria	139, 150
anus	119
anxiety	18, 136
anxiety disorder	17
anxiety neurosis	18
aorta (aortae)	118
aortic aneurysm	149
aortography	157
apex cordis	118
Apgar score	10, 13
aphasia	136
apnea	167
appendicitis	149
appendix	119
apron	103
arm	113
armpit	113
armpit hair	113
armrest	67
aroma therapy	174
arrhythmia	138, 149, 167
art therapy	174
artery	168
arthritis	147
arthrography	156
artificial arm	66
artificial hand	66
artificial insemination	21
artificial larynx	6
artificial leg	66

artificial limb	6
artificial respiration	171
artificial teeth	66
as necessary	92
ascending colon	119
asphyxia	23
aspiration	39
aspirator	67
assessment	55
Association for Welfare of the Mentally and Physically Disabled	52
asthma	148
astigmatism	150
at bedtime	93
ataxia	136
athlete's foot	151
atopic dermatitis	11, 151
attack	10
attention deficit hyperactivity disorder	12
audiometer	162
auditory hallucination	136
auditory tube	121
auricle	120
auscultation	166
autism	18
automated external defibrillator	6
autonomy	3
autopsy	42
average life expectancy	54
avian flu	153

B

babbling	13
baby bottle	14, 24
baby boy	13
baby food	14, 25
baby girl	13
baby talk	13
baby tooth	121
back	113
back of the hand	113
back tooth	121
backache	136
bacteria culture	156
bad breath	141
balance	69
baldness	141
Band-Aid	65
bandage	65
bankruptcy	7
barbershop	64
barely tolerable	142
bargaining	41
barium enema	157
basal body temperature	22
Basedow's disease	152
Basic Disability Pension	52
basic life support	171
basin	68
basket	64
bath	101
bath towel	101
bathrobe	64
bathroom	62
bathtub	102
bearable	142
bed bath	101
bedclothes	103
bedding	64
bedpan	67, 102
bedrail	64
bedridden elderly	38
bedside table	64
bedsore	40, 141
bedwetting	11
bee sting	135
before meals	92
behavior therapy	174
behavioral and psychological symptoms of dementia	39
belly	113
belly button	113
benign	7
biceps jerk	169
bidet	64
bifocals	66
big toe	114
bile duct calculus	149
biochemical examination of blood	160
biopsy	155
bipolar disorder	17
birth canal	23
birth control	22
birth control pills	22
birth rate	27

bis in die	92
bite	151
blanched	140
blanket	103
bleeding	135
bleeding time	161
blindness	151
blink	99
blister	141
blistered	140
bloating	138
blocked nose	139
blood clot	5
blood coagulation inhibitor	96
blood donation	51
blood lab	63
blood plasma	160
blood platelet	160
blood pressure	155, 167
blood pressure gauge	67
blood product	51
blood sample	159
blood sample holder	67
blood sedimentation rate	160
blood serum	160
blood sugar test	159
blood transfusion	3, 171
blood type	159
blood vessel	118
blood volume	159
bloodshot eyes	139
bloody stool	138
bloody urine	139
blow one's nose	99
blurred vision	140
body fat percentage	34
body mass index	4, 34
body odor	141, 151, 168
body surface area	168
body temperature	167
boil	141
boiling water	65
bonding	13
bone	116
bone and joint	169
bone marrow	122
bone-marrow bank	51
bottle feeding	14
bowel movements	102

bowel sound	169
bowl	100
brace	66
brace wearing	6
bradycardia	138, 167
braille writer	6
brain	117
brain concussion	148
brain death	3, 40
brain surgery	172
brain tumor	12, 148
brainstem	117
brassiere	103
bread	100
breakfast	99
breakup of a family	34
breakup of one's marriage	7
breakup with a lover	6
breast	113
breast binder	14
breast cancer	26
breast feeding	14
breast milk	14
breast pump	24
breastbone	116
breath sound	169
breathing difficulty	137
breech presentation	23
bronchitis	148
bronchoconstrictor	95
bronchodilator	95
bronchoscope	162
bronchoscopy	156
bronchus (bronchi)	118
bruise	151
brushing	101
bulimia nervosa	17
bullying	34
bump	151
burn	151
burning pain	143
burnout	41
burp	99, 138
buttocks	113
button	103

C

Caesarean section	24
café	64
cafeteria	64

calcium	160
calf	114
call bell	64
call button	64
campaign to prevent from becoming bedridden	38
cancer nursing	2, 38, 57
cane	67
canine tooth	121
canker sore	141
capillary	118
capsule	94
carcinostatic	96
cardiac catheterization	157
cardiac death	40
cardiac diet	100
cardiac murmur	168
cardiac surgery	172
cardiologist	83
cardiology	83
cardiomyopathy	148
cardiopulmonary resuscitation	13
cardiorespiratory	167
cardiotonic agent	96
care equipment	46
care insurance	45
care manager	45
care of a family member	40
care plan	46
care support	45
caregiver	45
carpus (carpi)	116
cart	100
caseworker	45
cashier	63, 83
cast	67
cast immobilization	6
casualty	42
cataract	150
catheter	162
catheter infection	5
catheter obstruction	4
catheterization	4, 172
cavity	152
cavography	157
cecum (ceca)	119
cell phone	104
Celsius	167
census	54
centigrade	167
cerebellum	117
cerebral anemia	148
cerebral infarction	147
cerebral paralysis	25
cerebral thrombosis	147
cerebrospinal fluid examination	156
cerebrum	117
certified health food	3
certified social worker	2
cervical	169
cervical canal	26
cervical cancer	25
cervical vertebra	116
change of pace	40
chap	152
charge nurse	81
cheating	7
cheek	112
chemotherapy	5, 173
chest	113, 167
chest binder	65
chest circumference	168
chest pain	137
chest X-ray	155
chew	99
Cheyne-Strokes respiration	137
chickenpox	11
chief administrator	81
child abuse	34
child guidance center	35
child welfare	35
child-rearing allowance	35
childbirth	7, 23
childhood bronchial asthma	12
childhood cancer	12
Children's Charter	35
children's home	35
chills	134
chin	112
Chinese herbal medicine	93
chiropractic	174
chloride	160
cholecystitis	149
cholera	152
cholesterol-lowering agent	96
choluria	150
chopsticks	100

chromosomal aberration	25
chronic	142
chronic disease	5
chronotherapy	174
clamp	66
clavicle	116
clavus	152
cleansing cream	101
cleft lip	12
cleft palate	12
clerk	83
climatotherapy	173
clinic	32, 51
clinical engineer	2
clinical laboratory	51
clinical nurse specialist	81
clinical nursing	58
clinical nutrition	3
clinical psychologist	2, 82
clothing	103
coagulation time	161
coccyx (coccyges)	116
codependency	16
cognitive behavioral therapy	18
cognitive function decline	38
cognitive therapy	173
coil	22
coin laundry	62
cold medicine	95
cold sweat	135
colic	11
colitis	149
collagenosis	152
collar bone	116
colon cancer	149
colonoscopy	157
color Doppler echocardiography	157
color perception test	158
color therapy	174
colostrum	25
coma	137
comfort measures	42
comforter	64
commode	68, 102
community health nursing	56
community medical examinations	32
complementary therapy	173
complete blood count	160
complication	5
comprehensive geriatric assessment	37
compress	172
compressed air outlet	67
computerized axial tomography	155
computerized tomography scan	155
concha of auricle	120
conference	3
conflict	19
confusion	134
congenital	7
congenital esophageal atresia	12
congenital hip dislocation	12
congestion	138
conjunctiva	120
conjunctivitis	151
consent form	104
constipation	5, 138
consultation room	62
contact lenses	103
contagious	53
contagious disease	5
contagious disease ward	62
container	162
contaminated	53
continuous	142
contraception	22
contraceptive	22
contrast medium	162
control therapy	172
contusion	151
convulsion	134
cool	140
core symptom	39
cornea	120
coronary artery	118
coronary artery disease	148
coronary care unit	63
corset	67
cortisone-glucose tolerance test	159
cosmetic surgery	172
cotton balls	65
cotton swab	65
cough	134

cough medicine	95
cough syrup	95
coughing fits	134
Council on Public Health	51
counseling	3
counselor	33
countermeasure against cancer	51
counting fingers	169
cracked	140
cramp	147
crampy pain	143
cranial nerve	169
crash cart	68
crawl	13
cream	94
creatinine	161
critical care nursing	57
critical path method	55
crown	66
crowning	24
crackle	137
crust	141
crutch (crutches)	67
CTスキャン	155
cuddle	13
cuff	67
Cumulative Index for Nursing and Allied Health Literature	56
cup	162
Cushing's disease	152
cut	151
cyanosis	3, 134
cystitis	149
cyto-toxic	96
cytomegalovirus infection	26
cytotechnology	156

D

daily activity center for elderly	37
daily living training center	17
dandruff	141
day service	37
death and dying	41
death certificate	41
death education	41
death instinct	41
death of a close relative	40
death of a family member	40
death of one's child	7
death of one's spouse	40
death rate	27
death rattle	41
death spots	42
death struggle	41
death with dignity	40
deathwatch	38, 41
debt	6
decayed tooth	152
decubitus ulcer	141
deep tendon reflex	169
defecation reflex	11
defibrillator	67
degree of aging	38
dehydration	5, 13, 134
delayed puberty	33
delirium	5, 137
delivery room	23, 63
delivery table	23
dementia	18, 38
dementia with Lewy bodies	38
dengue fever	153
denial	41
dental caries	152
dental hygienist	82
dental technician	83
dentist	84
dentistry	84
dentures	66, 103
dependence	16
dependence on medical care	33
depilation	3
depression	17, 41
dermatologist	84
dermatology	84
dermis	121
descending colon	119
despair	41
detergent	102
detoxication	171
development of fetus	10
developmental disorder	17
developmental nursing	10
dexter	166
diabetes	152
diabetic diet	100
diagnosis related group	55
diagnostic scheme	55

dialysis	172
diaper	38
diaper rash	13
diaphragm	22, 118
diarrhea	5, 138, 149
diastolic blood pressure	168
diet therapy	173
dietary guidelines	35
dietetic treatment	6
dietitian	82
difficulty in hearing	139
difficulty in urinating	139
digestive	95
digestive medicine	95
dignity	39
dilation and curettage	26
dilation of the pupil	140
dining room	64
dioxin	53
diplopia	151
direct bilirubin	161
director of nursing department	81
disability support services center	17
disaster	53
disaster countermeasure	53
disaster nursing	2
discharge	135
discharge guidance	4
discharge support	4, 32
discomfort	19
disease prevention	32
dish	100
disinfectant	65
disinfectant cotton	65
disinterest	41
dislocation	147
disorder	5
disorientation	136
disposable diaper	66
disseminated intravascular coagulation	25
distilled water	65
distrust	41
disuse syndrome	39
diuretic	95
divorce	7
divorce rate	54
dizziness	134
DNA testing	156
DNA検査	156
do not resuscitate	41
doctor	82
doctor in charge	82
domestic violence	19, 34
Doppler ultrasonography	157
dorsal position	175
dorsal recumbent position	175
dosage	93
dose	93
Down's syndrome	12
doze off	99
drain tube	67
dream	99
dressing	65, 66, 104
dressing cart	68
drool	13, 99
drug abuse	17
drug dependence	19
drug tariff	50
drug therapy	173
drug therapy monitoring	4
dry	140
dry eye	139
dry mouth	135
dry skin	140, 151
dry throat	135
dryer	102
dull pain	143
duodenal ulcer	149
duodenum	119
during a meal	93
dustcloth	104
duvet	64
dysmenorrhea	21, 33
dysphagia	5
dyspnea	137
dysuria	150

E

ear	112
ear discharge	139
ear lobe	112
ear pain	139
ear, nose and throat specialist	84
eardrum	120
early adolescence	33

earwax	139
eating disorder	17
Ebola hemorrhagic fever	153
eclampsia	26
ectopic pregnancy	25
eczema	141
edema	135
educational plan	55
effacement	26
effective dose	93
elbow	113
elective abortion	22
electric blanket	64
electrical appliance	104
electrocardiogram	157
electroconvulsive therapy	174
electroencephalography	156
electromyography	156
electron microscope	162
elevator	63
eligibility	50
emaciation	34, 135
embryo	26
emergency buzzer	102
emergency care system	52
emergency evacuation route	53
emergency exit	62
emergency medical service	171
emergency medical technician	51, 83
emergency nursing	57
emergency shelter	53
emergency surgery	171
emergency ward	62
emesis	134
emetic	95
employed	7
employees' pension	50
empty nest	7
endocrinologist	83
endocrinology	83
endoscope	66, 162
endoscopic examination	157
endoscopic operation	172
endoscopy	157
endoscopy department	63
endstage	38
enema	3, 68, 172
energy-based therapy	174
engorgement	24
enteritis	149
entrance	35
environmental sanitation	53
epidermis	121
epidural block	24
epigastric distress	138
epiglottis	118
epilepsy	5, 148
episiotomy	26
episode	135, 142
erectile dysfunction	3
erythrocyte	122, 160
esophagoscopy	157
esophagus	119
estrogen	26
Eugenic Protection Act	24
euthanasia	40
evaluation	55
every	92
every day	92
every hour	92
every other day	92
every week	92
evidence-based healthcare	56
evidence-based medicine	56
evidence-based nursing	56
examination of the fundus	158
examination of the visual field	158
exanthema	141
excessive appetite	135
excessive urination	139
excitement	19
excoriated	140
excoriation	151
exercise	104
exercise therapy	173
expansive delusion	19
expected date of delivery	23
expectorant	95
expulsive force	23
external	166
external acoustic meatus	120
external ear	120
extirpative surgery	172
extremely low birth weight infant	10
eye	112

eye chart	162
eye doctor	84
eye irritation	140
eye matter	140
eye mucus	140
eye ocular movement	168
eye pain	139
eye patch	65
eye test	34, 158
eye tooth	121
eye-drops	94
eyeball	120
eyebrow	112
eyelash	112
eyelid	112

F

face	112
face presentation	23
face washing	101
facial neuralgia	148
Fahrenheit	167
failure in the entrance examination	34
failure to thrive	12
faint	40
faintness	136
fall prevention	38
fall risk evaluation	38
fallopian tube	26
false teeth	66, 103
family background	34
family breakdown	34
family discord	34
family disease	5
family doctor	45, 82
family medicine	83
family nursing	2, 57
family policy	35
family therapy	18, 174
fasting blood sugar	159
fasting hypoglycemia	158
fatty acid	161
faucet	102
fear	18
fear of other people	19
febrile convulsion	11
feces test	157
feeding tube	6
feeding tube diet	3
feeling of fatigue	135
feeling of helplessness	137
feeling of pressure in one's chest	137
feeling of weariness	135
feeling troubled	18
femur (femora)	116
ferrum	161
fertility drug	21
fertilized egg	21
fetal distress	10, 23
fetal heart rate	10
fetal monitoring	10
fetal therapy	26
fetus	10
fever	134
fiber bronchoscopy	156
fiberoptic endoscopy	158
fiberscope	162
fibrin and fibrinogen degradation product	161
fibrinogen	161
fibula	117
filter	69
filter paper	65
finger breadth	169
finger cot	65
finger nail	113
finger sucking	13
fire extinguisher	62
first aid	171
fit	10
five stages of dying	41
flashlight	69, 103
flower shop	64
flu	152
fluids	100
flushed	140
fontanelle	13
food administration	32
food allergy	11
food handlers	53
food poisoning	5, 149
food refusal	19
food sanitation	53
foot	114
foot bath	101
foot rail	64

foot-bath tub	69
footrest	67
forceps	66
forearm	113
forehead	112
forgetfulness	16
formula	14
foster care	35
foster parent	35
four times a day	92
Fowler's position	175
fracture	147
freckle	141
free fatty acid	161
frequent urination	139
frequently	142
fretfulness	18
frigidity	3
front tooth	121
frontotemporal dementia	38
frozen shoulder	147
frustration	136
full term birth	23
fundamental nursing	56
funeral arrangements	42
fuss	13

G

gallbladder	119
gallstones	149
garbage bag	104
gargle	95
gastric analysis	157
gastric fistula	4
gastric juice	119
gastric tube	68
gastric ulcer	149
gastritis	149
gastrocamera	162
gastroenteritis	153
gastroenterologist	83
gastroenterology	83
gastrofiberscopy	157
gastrointestinal endoscopy	157
gastroscopy	157
gastrostoma	4
gauge	162
gauze	65
gene therapy	173
general anesthesia	171
general diet	99
general hospital	51
general practice	32
general practitioner	82
general reception	63
general status	166
general ward	62
generalized pain	143
genetic testing	156
genital bleeding	25
genitals	114
geriatric depression scale	38
geriatric nursing	56
geriatric syndrome	39
gestational diabetes	25
get tired easily	135
gingiva	168
glass stick	162
glasses	103
glaucoma	150
Global Program on AIDS	54
globulin	160
glucose	160
glucose tolerance test	159
glucosuria	139
gnawing pain	143
go out	104
gonadotropic hormone	159
gonorrhea	153
goose bumps	141
gout	152
graduation	35
grandiose delusions	19
granule	94
grasp	13
grasping power	169
grief	19, 41
grief care	4, 39
griping pain	143
groin	113
group home	37
group therapy	174
growth curve	34
growth disorder	34
growth hormone	33, 158
growth hormone treatment	12
growth support	10
grudge	19

gruel	99
gum tissue	121
gums	121
gurney	67
gynecological checkup	21
gynecologist	84
gynecology	84

H

hair	112
hair brush	101
hair bulb	121
hair comb	101
hair root	121
haircut	101
hall	63
hallucination	136
hand	113
hand bath	101
hand dynamometer	162
hand motion	169
hangover	135
Hashimoto thyroiditis	152
hatred	19
hay fever	150
head	112
head circumference	168
head mirror	69
head nurse	81
headache	134
Health and Medical Service Act for the Aged	37
health and welfare policy	58
health assessment	3
health care benefit coverage	50
health inspector	53
health instruction	33
health insurance	50
health insurance card	104
health problem	38
health promotion	52
Health Promotion Act	52
health resort therapy	174
health statistics	2
healthcare facility for the elderly	37
healthy life expectancy	37
hearing aid	66
hearing test	34, 158
heart	118
heart attack	148
heart bypass operation	172
heart disease	148
heart failure	148
heart rate	168
heart sound	168
heartburn	138
heat rash	13, 141
heaviness	19
heaviness of the head	136
heavy feeling in the stomach	138
heel	114
height	168
help with bath	102
help with eating	100
help with falling sleep	103
help with shower	102
helper	45
hematinic	96
hematocrit	160
hematuria	139
hemiplegia	148
Hemoccult test	158
hemoglobin	160
hemophilia	152
hemoptysis	137
hemorrhage	135
hemostasis	171
hepatic cancer	149
hepatic stimulant	95
hepatitis	149, 153
herbal therapy	174
hereditary disease	5
heredity	26
herpes	153
hiccup	99
high blood pressure	138
high fever	167
high risk infant	10
high-protein diet	100
hircismus	151
histaminergic drug	96
HIV antibody test	156
HIVウイルス	153
HIV抗体テスト	156
hives	141
hoarseness	137
hold up one's head	13

Holter monitor	162
home care	46
home care nursing	57
home for fatherless families	35
home mechanical ventilation	46
home monitoring system	46
home nursing station	46
home oxygen therapy	46
home palliative treatment	45
home parenteral nutrition	46
home pregnancy test	21
home welfare measures	45
home-buying	7
home-care management	45
home-care management fee	46
home-care support center	46
home-care worker	45
home-delivery service	46
home-visit care	45
home-visit dietary instruction	45
home-visit nursing station	32
homeopathy	174
homicide	40
hopelessness	137
hora somni	93
hormonal drug	96
hormone replacement therapy	26
hormone therapy	173
horticulture therapy	173
hospice	40
hospital director	81
hospital gown	64
hospital infection	2
hospital room	62
hospital school	11
hot	140
hot flash	27, 135
hot-water bottle	66
hotline	46
household medicine	93
human chorionic gonadotropin	159
Human Genome Project	51
human immunodeficiency virus	153
human resource agency for welfare services	52
humerus (humeri)	116
hydration	100
hydrocephalus	12
hygiene	53
hyperglycemia	5
hyperpnea	167
hypertension	138
hyperventilation	167
hypnotic therapy	173
hypoglycemia	5
hypogonadism	12
hypophysis	122
hypotension	138
hypoventilation	167
hypoxia	168
hysteria	18

I

ice pack	66
ictus	10
ID card	104
ileum	119
illness of a family member	7
imminent abortion	25
immune therapy	173
immunization	13
Immunization Law	53
immunocompromised	152
immunological test	156
immunosuppressant	96
implantation	21
implementation	55
in vitro fertilization	21
incidence rate	54
incision	172
incisor	121
incontinence	38, 139
incubator	13
incurable disease	40
independence support	11, 16
index finger	113
individual therapy	174
induced pluripotent stem cell	122
industrial hygiene	2
infant	13
infant mortality rate	27
infection control	2
infection control nursing	57
infection management	2
infectious	53
infectious disease	32

Infectious Disease Prevention Act	54
infectious medical waste	53
infectious waste bin	67
inferior vena cava	118
inferior	166
infertility	25
influenza	152
information counter	63
information systems	54
informed consent	2
infrared therapy	173
inhalation	171
inhalent	94
inhaler	67
inherited disease	5
injection needle	6
insomnia	18
inspection	166
insulin	4, 46
insulin sensitivity test	159
insult	10
intellectually disabled	11
intense	142
intense self-consciousness	19
intensive care unit	63
inter cibos	92
intercostal	169
intercourse	21
intermittent fever	167
intermittent self-catheterization	11
internal	166
internal ear	121
internal examination	22
internal medicine	83
International Council of Nurses	56
internist	83
interpersonal psychotherapy	18
interprofessional collaboration	45
intestinal obstruction	149
intolerable	142
intoxication	134
intracerebral hemorrhage	147
intractable	142
intractable disease	5
intradermal injection	171
intramuscular injection	171
intraocular pressure measurement	158
intrauterine device	22
intrauterine growth restriction	25
intravenous drip	171
intravenous hyperalimentation	4
intravenous injection	171
intravenous injection pole	67
introduction to nursing	56
intubation	172
involution of the uterus	24
iodine tincture	96
iPS細胞	122
iris	120
irregular menstruation	33
irregular pulse	138
irreversible	142
irrigator	6, 67
irritability	135, 136
irritation	19
itch	140
itching	134
itching sensation	11
itchy eyes	140

J

jammed finger	136
Japan Medical Association	52
Japanese Nursing Association	56
Japanese Red Cross Society	52
jaundice	135
jaw	112
jejunum	119
jitteriness	136
job shortage	34
joint	117
joint pain	136

K

kalium	160
keratitis	151
ketone body	158
key person	45
kidney	119
kidney failure	150
kin	40
knee	114
knee-chest position	175
kneecap	117

L

knuckle	113
lab technician	82
labor pain	23
labor room	23
laboratory	63
laceration	151
lack of appetite	19
lactation	24
lancet	66
laparoscope	162
laparoscopic examination	157
laparoscopy	157
large baby	24
large intestine	119
larynx (larynges)	118
laser surgery	172
late childbearing	23
lateral	166
lateral position	175
latex gloves	65
laughter therapy	174
laundry	102
laundry bag	102
laundry room	62
lavatory	62
laxative	95
lead apron	162
learning disabilities	12
left	166
left atrium	118
left ventricle	118
leg	114
leg-rest	67
lens	120
letdown reflex	25
lethal dose	93
lethargy	41
leukemia	12, 152
leukocyte	122, 160
liaison nursing	57
libido	3
licensed practical nurse	81
life table	54
life-prolonging treatment	5
lifesaving drug	93
ligament	117
light sense	168
light therapy	173
lights-out time	103
line	141
lip	112
liquids	100
liquid diet	100
liquid medicine	94
listening	16, 39
lithotomy position	175
little finger	113
little toe	114
live birth	10
liver	119
liver cancer	149
liver cirrhosis	149
liver function test	157
living will	4
living-donor operation	172
lobby	63
local anesthesia	171
localized pain	143
location	166
locker	64
locomotive syndrome	46
loitering	38
loneliness	18, 40
loose bowel movements	138
loss	41, 135, 138
lost love	6
low birth weight	10
low blood pressure	138
low-salt diet	100
lower lid	112
lower lip	112
lozenge	94
lubricating topical anesthetic	4
lukewarm water	65
lumbago	136
lumbar vertebra	116
lumbar	169
lump	27, 141, 151
lumpectomy	172
lunch	99
lung	118
lung cancer	148
lunula	113
lymph	122
lymph gland	122
lymph node	122, 169

lymphocyte	122

M

macular degeneration	150
magic bullet	93
magnesium	160
magnetic resonance imaging	155
makeup	101
malaria	152
malignant	7
malignant lymphoma	152
malnutrition	5, 39
malpractice	2
mania	17
manic depression	17
manic state	19
marriage	7
marriage rate	54
massage therapy	173
mastitis	26
maternal and child health	24, 57
maternal and child health handbook	24
maternal management	24
maternal nursing	57
maternity blues	22
mattress	64
maximum dose	93
mealtime	99
mean	54
mean blood pressure	168
meaninglessness	41
measles	11
measures for infectious disease control	53
measuring cup	68
measuring spoon	68
measuring tape	68
meconium	24
medical assistance program	50
medical care benefit	50
medical care in sparsely populated areas	32
medical care plan	50
medical center	51
medical checkup	13
medical insurance system	45
medical insurance system for the elderly aged 75 or over	37, 45
medical policy	2
Medical Practitioners' Act	52
medical social worker	45, 82
medical sociology	57
medical supplies	67
medical therapy	173
Medical Treatment and Supervision Act	17
medication	173
medication cart	68
megalomania	19
melanin blocker	96
melanoma	151
memory loss	136
meninx (meninges)	117
menopausal disorder	26
menopause	26
menorrhagia	22
menstrual cramps	22
menstrual disorder	22
menstrual pain	22
menstruate	21
mental care	16
mental disease	17
mental health	3, 16
Mental Health Act	16
mental health center	51
mental therapy	173
mentally challenged person	16
mercy killing	40
metabolic syndrome	3
metacarpal	116
metallic items	103
metatarsal	117
metrorrhagia	25
microscope	162
mid line	169
middle ear	120
middle finger	113
midwife	22, 82
midwifery	56
migraine	136
mild	142
mild cognitive impairment	39
mild pain	143
miliaria	141
milk secretion	24
Ministry of Health, Labour and Welfare	51

miscarriage	23
miss one's period	21
moderate	142
moisturizer	11
molar	121
mole	141
monitor	68
mood disorder	17
mood swings	136
morbidity	54
morning sickness	23
mortgage	6
mortuary	64
mosquito bite	135
mother-to-be	21
mother-to-child transmission	22
mottled	140
mouth	112
mouth ulcer	141
mouthwash	95
moving	7
MRI technician	82
MRI技師	82
mucus	137
multimodal treatment	6
multiple	7
multiple pregnancy	25
mumps	11
municipal health center	51
murder	40
muscle	117
muscle pain	136
muscle relaxer	96
muscle spasm	136
music therapist	82
music therapy	174
mydriasis	151
myelography	156
myocardial infarction	148
myocarditis	148
myopia	151
myosis	151

N

nail bed	113
nailclipper	101
nap	103
nape of neck	112
nasal cavity	121
nasal discharge	139
nasal septum	121
naso-gastric tube	68
nasogastric tube feeding	4
National Disaster Act	53
national health insurance	45
national hospital	51
national hospital organization	51
natural death	40
natural killer cell	122
nausea	134
navel	113
nebulizer	68
neck	112
needle for injection	66
negative	167
neglect	19
neonatal behavioral assessment scale	10
neonatal hypoglycemia	12
neonatal intensive care unit	10
neonatal period	24
neonate	10
nephritis	149
nephrosis	150
nerve	117, 169
nervous breakdown	17
nervousness	136
neuralgia	148
neurologist	84
neurology	84
neurosis	18
neurosurgeon	83
neurosurgery	83
neurotropic drug	17
never	142
newborn resuscitation	13
next of kin	40
nidation	21
night nurse	81
night sweat	135
nipple	113
nipple of baby bottle	14
no problem	166
nocturia	150
noninvasive positive pressure ventilation	4
normal birth	23
normal saline	94

Norovirus	153
nose	112
nose drops	94
nosebleed	139
nostril	112
'not myself'	135
nothing particular	166
nuchal translucency	22
number	166
numbness	136
numero	166
nurse practitiner	81
nurse's aid	82
nurse's license	52
nursery	63
nurses' station	62
nursing administration	57
nursing arts	58
nursing assistant	82
nursing audit committee	56
nursing care benefit	46
nursing care plan	55
nursing diagnosis	55
nursing education	57
nursing ethics	58
nursing home	32
nursing informatics	56
nursing interview	55
nursing practice	58
nursing process	55
nursing research	57
nursing research methodology	57
nursing science	56
nursing service delivery system	58
nursing skills	58
nursing sociology	57
nursing theory	56
nurture	10
nutritional guidance	32
nutritional supplement	93
nutritionist	82

O

obesity	135
objective data	55
oblique	166
obstetric shock	23
obstetrician	84
obstetrics	84
occasionally	142
occupational health nursing	57
occupational therapist	82
occupational therapy	173
occupied	102
oiled paper	65
ointment	94
oliguria	139, 150
omni hora	92
once a day	92
oncology nursing	57
operating room	62
operating room nursing	57
operating table	68
ophthalmic examination	158
ophthalmologist	84
ophthalmology	84
ophthalmoscope	162
optic nerve	117
oral care	6
oral glucose tolerance test	159
oral rehydration therapy	172
orderly	82
organ donation	52
Organ Transplant Law	52
organ transplantation	3, 172
orthodontics	84
orthodontist	84
orthopedics	83
orthopedist	83
orthoptist	82
osteoporosis	39, 147
otitis media	150
otorhinolaryngologist	84
otorhinolaryngology	84
outbreak	33
outcast	34
outlet	68
outpatient nursing	2
outpatient surgery	172
outpatient therapy	51
outpatient window	63
ovary	120
over dose	93
over the bed table	64
over-the-counter medicine	93
overeating	19
ovulation	21

oxygen mask	66
oxygen outlet	64
oxygen tank	68

P

pacemaker	174
pain	134
pain in the nose	139
pain management	3, 42
painful intercourse	21
painful urination	139
painkiller	42, 95
pajamas	103
pale	140
palliation	41
palliative care	38, 41
palliative operation	172
palliative treatment	41, 173
palm	113
palpitation	137, 166
pancreas	119
pancreatitis	149
panic	19
Papanicolaou smear test	22
paralysis	136
paramedic	2, 83
parasite	53, 158
parasympathetic nerve	117
parathyroid gland	122
parenting support	24
parents' divorce	34
Parkinson's disease	5, 39
paroxysm	10, 134
parrot fever	153
partial thromboplastin time	161
pass away	40
pass gas	99
patella (patellae)	117
patellar tendon reflex	169
pathology examination	156
patient survey	54
patient-nurse interaction	55
patient's copayment system	50
patients' lounge	62
pediatric nursing	56
pediatrician	84
pediatrics	84
pelvic bone	116
pelvis	26, 116

penis	120
perinatal center	63
perinatal mortality rate	54
perinatal period	23
period	21
peripheral nerve	117
peritoneal dialysis	4
peritonitis	149
permanent tooth	121
persistent	142
pertussis	11
PET technician	82
PET技師	82
Petri dish	66
phalanx (phalanges)	116
pharmacist	82
pharmacy	63, 93
pharynx (pharynges)	118
phlegm	137
phonocardiography	157
phospholipid	161
photophobia	148
photosensitivity	140, 148
physical assessment	3
physical checkup	155
physical examination	155
physical therapist	82
physical therapy	173
physically disabled person	52
physician	82
physician in charge	82
physiological function test	155
physiological lab department	63
pill	94
pillow	103
pineal gland	122
pinky	113
pitcher	69
pituitary gland	122
placebo	93
placenta	26, 120
placenta previa	24
plan	55
planning	55
plaque	141
plasma	122
plaster	94
plastic pad	65
plastic surgeon	84

plastic surgery	84, 172
platelet	122
play room	62
play therapy	174
pneumonia	148
pneumothorax	148
poison control center	54
poisoning	134
polio	11
pollinosis	150
pollution	53
polyp	135
polyuria	139, 150
population	54
pore	121
portable oxygen bottle	46
portable toilet	68
portable transfusion system	46
position change	38
positioning aids	6
positive	167
positron emission tomography	155
post cibos	92
post cibum	92
post operative diet	100
post traumatic stress disorder	18
postnatal depression	26
postpartum blues	22
potassium	160
powder	94
powdered medicine	94
pre-eclampsia	25
precocious puberty	33
prednisolone-glucose tolerance test	159
pregnancy	7, 21
pregnancy induced hypertension	25
pregnancy test	21
premature baby	13
premature delivery	23
premenstrual syndrome	21
preparation for eating	100
preparation for sleeping	103
prescription	93
present condition	166
pressure bandage	66
prevalence rate	54
preventive medicine	2, 93
prickling pain	143
primary care	2, 51
primary health care nursing	57
primary nurse	81
primary nursing	55
primary physician	82
primitive reflex	11
private room	62
pro re nata	92
problem-based learning	56
proctoscope	162
prodromal period	16
progesterone	26
progress notes	55
projection of supply and demand for nursing personnel	52
prolactin	159
promotion	7
prone position	175
prostate cancer	150
prostate gland	120
prosthesis	66
protection of privacy	4
protective shield	162
protein bound iodine	159
prothrombin time	161
pruritus	134
psychiatric nursing	56
psychiatric pharmacotherapy	18
psychiatric social worker	2
psychiatric-liaison nursing	57
psychiatrist	84
psychiatry	84
psychogenic	16
psychological care	39
psychological first aid	18
psychological therapy	173
psychosomatic disorder	18
psychotropic drug	17
public funding	50
public health	32, 53
public health center	32, 51, 53
public health nurse	32, 53
Public Health Service Act	54
puerperal period	23
pulmonary emphysema	148
pulmonary function test	156
pulmonologist	83

pulmonology	83
pulse	134
pulse oximeter	6, 46
pulse pressure	168
pulse	167
pupil	120
pupillary reflex	158
purpose in life	39
pus	140
push	23
pyelitis	150
pyorrhea	152
pyrexia	134
pyuria	150

Q

Q-tip	65
quality control	55
quality of life	55
quaque	92
quaque die	92
quarantine	53
quarter in die	92
quick pulse	167
quilt	64
quisque	92

R

rabies	153
radiation therapy	5,172
radical operation	172
radical treatment	174
radiograph	155
radiography department	63
radiologist	83
radiology	83
radius (radii)	116
rale	137
rapid pulse	138
rash	141
razor	101
reason for being	39
receptionist	83
recovery room	63
recreation therapy	174
rectal cancer	149
rectal examination	23
rectum	119
recumbent position	175

recurrent miscarriage	25
recurring	142
red	140
red blood cell	122, 160
red blood count	160
red eyes	139
reddened	140
reflex	169
reflexology	174
refrigerator	64
regenerative therapy	173
regional comprehensive care	32
regional health and medical care plan	51
regional medical cooperation system	32
registered nurse	81
registration	63
regression	19
rehabilitation center	63
relaxation	4
relief technique	2
remarriage	7
remittent fever	167
renal disease diet	100
renal function test	158
repeat a grade in school	34
reproductive health	21
requiring care	38
resident	82
respiration	134, 168
respirator	68
respiratory distress syndrome	11
respiratory management	46
respiratory medicine	83
respiratory rate	168
respiratory sound	169
respite care	42, 46
restroom	62
restructuring	6
resuscitation	2
retina	120
retinopathy	150
retirement	7
return to school	33
reversible	142
rheumatism	147
rheumatoid arthritis	147
rheumatoid arthritis test	156

rhinitis	150
rib	116
rib cage	113
rice	99
right atrium	118
right of self-determination	3
right ventricle	118
right	166
rigidity	135
rigor mortis	42
ring finger	113
ring shaped cushion	68
ringing in one's ears	139
roseola	141
rotation	23
rough	140
rubber glove	65
rubbing alcohol	96
rubbish bin	64
rubella	11
runny eye	139
runny nose	134

S

sacral	169
sacrum (sacra)	116
sadness	41
saline	94
saliva	119, 141
salt-free diet	100
sample	54
sand play therapy	173
sanitary napkin	22
sanitary pad	22
sanitation inspector	53
sarcopenia	39
scale	69
scalpel	66
scaly	140
scapula (scapulae)	116
scar	141
schizophrenia	17
school counseling	33
school environmental health	33
school for children with disabilities	11
school health	57
school nurse	11
school nurs's office	33
school physical examination	33
sciatic nerve	117
sclera (scleras, sclerae)	120
scrape	151
scraped	140
scratch	151
screening study	155
scrub nurse	81
seasoning	100
sebaceous gland	121
second opinion	3
secondary sex characteristics	33
security blanket	14
sedation	39
sedative	17
seizure	10
seldom	142
self-care	46
self-catheterization	4
self-denial	41
self-disgust	41
self-esteem	19, 39
self-injection	46
self-injury	16
self-respect	39
semi-Fowler position	175
semissem	93
senile dementia	38
senile dementia center	37
senile pneumonia	39
senior citizens' club	37
sensation of stomach pressure	138
sense of defeat	41
sense of security	39
separandum	93
separation	7
sequela	5
serological test	160
Services and Support for people with Disabilities Act	16
setting for meal	100
severe	142
severe acute respiratory syndrome	153
severe pain	142
sewage treatment facility	54
sex education	33
sexual debility	3

sexual impotence	3
sexually transmitted disease	34, 153
shadow	137
shampoo	101
shampoo cart	68
sharp pain	142
shaver	101
shaving	101
shaving foam	101
shaving hair	172
sheet	64, 103
shin	114
shivering	13, 134
short stay	37
shortness of breath	169
shot	13
shoulder	112
shoulder blade	116
shower cap	101
shower room	62
side	113
side effect	93
sigmoid colon	119
sign	166
simplified menopausal index	26
Sims' position	175
sinister	166
Sister	81
sitting position	175
skin cancer	151
skin eruption	140
skin lotion	101
skin roughness	140
skull	116
sleeping pill	17
sleeplessness	19
slight	142
slight fever	167
slight pain	143
slightly	167
sling	66
slipped disk	136
slippers	103
slow pulse	138, 167
slurred speech	135
small forceps	66
small intestine	119
smoke alarm	62
snack between meals	100
sneeze	137
soap	101
SOAP charting	55
social and therapeutic horticulture	173
social isolation	19
social rehabilitation	46
social welfare	52
social withdrawal	16
sodium	160
soft	140
soft diet	100
soft spot	13
sole	114
solid diet	100
solution	94
sometimes	142
sore throat	134
soreness	134, 143
soul	40
spa therapy	173
special diet	99
special nursing home	37
specific gravity	158
speech therapist	82
speech therapy	173
sphincter	117
sphygmomanometer	67
spinal cord	117
spine	116
spirit	40
spiritual well-being	42
spirometry	156, 162
spittoon	68
splash guard	65
spleen	122
splint	67
sponge-bath	101
spoonful	93
sporadic	142
sprain	147
spray	94
sputum	137
sputum examination	155
squeezing pain	143
stab	151
stadiometer	34, 69
stairs	63

standing position	175
starting a business	7
starvation	40
stay out overnight	104
steam inhaler	68
sternum	116
steroid	11, 96
stethoscope	68, 162
stick	67
stiff shoulder	136
stiffness	134
stillbirth	23
stinging pain	143
stitch	143
stoma	4
stomach	119
stomach cramp	149
stomach tube	68
stomachache	138
stool	102
stool extraction	172
stool test	157
store	64
strabismus	151
stress	18
stress incontinence	139
stress test	156
stretch	99
stretcher	67
stroke	10, 147
student nurse	82
stuffy nose	139
stutter	135
sty	151
styling	101
subarachnoid hemorrhage	147
subchorionic hematoma	25
subcutaneous injection	171
subcutaneous tissue	121
subjective data	55
sublingual medication	94
suction	38, 46, 171
suction machine	68
sudden death	40
sudden infant death syndrome	12
suffocation	40
sugar-free diet	100
suicidal ideation	16
suicidal wishes	16
suicide	16, 40
suicide attempt	16
sun bathe	104
super-aged society	37
superior vena cava	118
superior	166
supervisor	81
supination	175
supine position	175
supper	99
supportive presence	39
suppository	3, 94
surgeon	83
surgery	83, 171
surgical gown	65
surgical nurse	81
surgical nursing	57
surgical theater	62
surgical therapy	173
surveillance system for tuberculosis and infectious diseases	53
suspension from school	35
suture	172
swallow	99
swallowing difficulty	39
sweat	99
sweat gland	121
swelling	135
swine flu	153
sympathetic nerve	117
symptom	166
symptomatic therapy	172
syndrome	166
syphilis	153
syringe	6, 66, 68
syrup	94
systolic blood pressure	167
S状結腸	119

T

T bandage	24
T lymphocyte	122
T-cell	122
tablet	94
tachycardia	138, 167
take a nap	99
talk in one's sleep	99
tampon	22, 65

tarsus (tarsi)	117
tartar	152
taste buds	119
taxi stand	64
team medical care	33
tear duct	120
teary eye	139
teething	13
telephone order	55
temperature	155
temple	112
temporary cancellation of classes	33
temporary childcare services	35
tendon	117
tendon reflex	156
tendovaginitis	147
tenosynovitis	147
tension	137
ter in die	92
terminal care	37
terminal stage	40
test for ova	158
test tube	66
testicle	120
the purpose of one's existence	39
the subjective well-being inventory	155
therapeutic diet	100
therapeutic plan	55
therapeutic touch	174
thermal therapy	173
thermometer	68
thigh	114
thoracic vertebra	116
thoracic	169
thorax	113
threat	18
three times a day	92
three-year-old infant check-up	35
throat	118
throbbing pain	143
thrombin time	161
thrombo test	161
thumb	113
thymus gland	122
thyroid gland	122
thyroid-stimulating hormone	158
tibia (tibiae)	117
timidity	137
tissue	102
tissue thromboplastin inhabitation test	161
to be held back	34
toe	114
toenail	114
toilet	62, 102
toilet paper	102
toilet training	11
toiletries	101
tongue	119
tongue depressor	66
tonsil	118
tonsillitis	150
tooth (teeth)	121
tooth brushing	101
tooth pick	100
toothache	141
toothbrush	101
toothpaste	101
top of the foot	114
topical medicine	96
total bilirubin	161
total cholesterol	161
total pain	4
total parenteral nutrition	4
total protein	160
tourniquet	67
towel	101
toxemia of pregnancy	25
toy	14
trachea (tracheae)	118
tracheostomy	6
trachoma	150
traffic accident	7
training benefit	46
tranquilizer	17
transfer of schools	35
transient ischemic attack	148
transverse colon	119
trash box	104
traumatic experience	19
tray	68, 100
treadmill test	157
treatment room	62
treatment table	68
treatment with hot baths	173

tremor	137
Trendelenburg's position	175
triage	3, 51
trigeminal nerve	117
triglyceride	161
trimester	23
trouble between one's wife and one's mother	35
trouble with superiors	6
truancy	33
truss	68
tub bath	24
tube feeding	3, 100
tube stand	68
tuberculin reaction	11
tuberculosis	148
tummy	113
tuning fork	162
Turner's syndrome	12
twice a day	92
twinge	141
T細胞	122
T字帯	24

U

ulna (ulnae)	116
ultrasonography	155
ultrasound	22
umbilical cord	24
umbilicus	113
unbearable	142
underachiever	34
underwear	103
uneasiness	136
unemployed	7
unemployment	6
unfaithfulness	7
universal health insurance coverage	50
upper arm	113
upper lid	112
upper lip	112
urea nitrogen	160
ureter	119
urethra	119
uric acid	161
urinal	68
urinalysis	158
urinary bladder	119
urinary stone	150
urinary tract infection	150
urinary urgency	139
urination	102
urine	102
urine bottle	68
urine test	158
urobilinogen	158
urologist	84
urology	84
urticaria	141, 152
uterine cancer	25
uterine myoma	25
uterus	26, 120
uvula	118

V

vaccination	13, 33
vaccine	93
vacuum extraction	24
vacuum extraction tube system	67
vagina	26, 120
vaginal discharge	22
vaginal examination	22
vaginitis	25
valuables	103
valve	118
varicella	11
vascular dementia	38
vasoconstrictor	96
vasodilator	96
vegetarian	100
vein	168
vending machine	62
ventilator	68
vertigo	137
vice director	81
victim	42
viral hepatitis	153
visiting	4
visiting care	32
visiting hours	104
visiting nurse	82
visiting nursing	57
visitor	104
visual acuity	168
visual field	168
vital signs	3

vital statistics	54
vitamin drops	93
vitamin K deficiency	26
vitreous body	120
vocal cords	118
vocational aid center	17
volunteer	83
volvulus	149
vomiting	134
vomiting blood	138

W

wafer	93
wagon	100
waist	113
waiting area	63
waiting room	63
wake-up time	103
walker	6
walker with brakes	67
warm	140
wart	152
wash-basin	101
wastebasket	64
water breaking	23
water utility	54
water	94
weakness	134
weight	168
weight gain	10
weight scale	34, 69
welfare	37
welfare commissioner	51
welfare facility of social insurance	52
welfare state	52
well-baby clinic	13
West Nile fever	153
wet	140

wheelchair	6, 67
wheezing	137
when hungry	93
whiplash injury	147
white blood cell	122, 160
wig	103
window shade	64
wisdom tooth	121
with meals	93
withdrawal of life support system	42
womb	120
women's health	58
World Health Organization	50
wrinkle	141
wrist	113
written order	55

X・Y

X-ray apparatus	162
X-ray department	63
X-ray examination	155
X-ray technician	82
X線技師	82
X線検査	155
X線撮影装置	162
X線体軸断層撮影法	155
yawn	99

その他

1時間ごと	92
1次救命処置	171
1日1回	92
1日2回	92
1日3回	92
1日4回	92
2次救命処置	171
3カ月の期間	23
3歳児健診	35

Index

略語

A	55, 166, 168	CE	2	G	168
abd	113, 167	CF	169	GA	157
a.c.	92	CGTT	159	GB	119
AC	168	CI	160	GDS	38
ACTH	159	CINAHL	56	GH	33, 158
add	167	CN	169	Glob	160
ADH	159	CNS	81	Glu	160
ADHD	12	CP	25, 137	GP	82, 169
AED	6	CPM	55	GTH	159
A/G ratio	160	CPR	13	GTT	159
AIDS	153	CR	167	GU	149
AJ	169	Crea	161	Hb	160
Alb	160	CSF exam.	156	HBP	138
ALD, Ald	159	CT	155, 161	HC	168
ALL	12	d	166	HCG, hCG	159
ALS	5, 171	D&C	26	Hct	160
aPTT	161	DBil	161	HGP	51
aq.	94	DBP	168	HIV	153
AT	174	dext	166	HM	169
ATR	169	DIC	25	HMV	46
B&J	169	DLB	38	HOT	46
BB	101	DNR	41	HPN	46
BBT	22	dos.	93	HR	168
BE	157	DRG	55	HRT	26
b.i.d.	92	DTR	169	h.s.	93
BJ	169	DU	149	HS	168
BLS	171	DV	19	Ht	168
BMI	4, 34	E	172	i.c.	92
BO	168	EBHC	56	IC	169
BP	155, 160, 167	EBM	56	ICN	56
BPSD	39	EBN	56	ICU	63
bra	103, 167	ECG	157	inf	166
BS	160, 169	ED	3, 93	int	166
BSA	168	EEG	156	IPPA	166
BSR	160	EKG	157	iPS cell	122
BT	161, 167, 174	EMG	156	IPT	18
BV	159	EMS	171	IUD	22
Bx	155	EMT	51, 83	IUGR	25
C	169	ENT	84	IV	6, 68, 171
C-section	24	EOM	168	IVF	21
Ca	160	ext	166	IVH	4
Cap	94	FA	161	JMA	52
CAT	155	FB	101, 169	JNA	56
cat.	150	Fbg	161	K	160
CBC	160	FBS	159	L	166, 169
CC	168	FDP	161	LA	118
CCU	63	Fe	161	lat	166
		FFA	161	LBP	138
		fx	147	LBW	10

LD	12, 93	PFA	18	SMI	26
LFT	157	PFT	156	SOB	169
LN	169	PGTT	159	sol	94
LPN	81	PIH	25	ss	93
LS	168	PL	161	ST	173
LV	118	Plat	160	STD	34, 153
MBP	168	PMS	21	STH	173
MCH	24	Pos	167	SUBI	155
MCI	39	PP	168	sup	166
Mg	160	PRL	159	supp	94
MI	148	p.r.n.	92	syr	94
ML	169	PT	82, 161	Tab	94
MRI	155	PTR	169	TB	148
N	169	PTSD	18	TBil	161
Na	160	PTT	161	TBT	161
NBAS	10	q, Q	92	TC	161
ND	55	QC	55	TCT	174
Neg	167	q.d.	92	TG	161
NH3	160	q.d.s.	92	Th	169
NI	55	QOD	92	TIA	148
NICU	10	QOL	55	t.i.d.	92
NK cell	122	QW	92	TP	160
No	166	R	166, 168	TPN	4
np	166	RA	118, 147	TR	11
NP	81	RA test	156	TSH	158
NPPV	4	RBC	160	TT	161
NS	94	RDS	11	TTIT	161
NT	22	ref	169	U	158
O	55	RN	81	UA	158, 161
OB	166	RR	168	Urea-N	160
OD	93	RS	169	US	155
OGTT	159	RT	172	V	168
Oh	92	RV	118	VA	168
oit	94	Rx	93	VE	24
OR	62	S	55, 137, 169	VF	168
ORT	172	s.	166	VS	3
OT	82	SAH	147	WBC	13, 160
OTC	93	SARS	153	WC	67
P	55, 167	SBP	167	WHO	50
PBI	159	SED	160	Wt	168
PBL	56	SG	158	X-P	155
p.c.	92	SIDS	12	°C	167
PD	4	sin	166	°F	167
PET	155	SL	167		

参考文献

看護行為用語分類（日本看護科学学会看護学学術用語検討委員会，編），日本看護協会出版会，2005.
ナースに必要な日常表現と略語第 2 版（助川尚子，他，著），医学書院，1996.
ICNP（看護実践国際分類），（国際看護協会編），日本看護協会出版会，2006.
N ANDA 看護診断定義と分類 2005 － 2006（日本看護診断学会，監訳，中木高夫，訳），医学書院，2005.
カルテ用語辞典 第 5 版 (大井静雄，編)，照林社，2014.
早引き看護・カルテ用語辞典【第 2 版】（飯田恭子，著），ナツメ社，2008.
外国で病気になったときあなたを救う本［第 5 版］（櫻井健司，監修），The Japan Times，2010.
看護・医学事典 第 7 版増補版 (井部 俊子，著)，医学書院 ,2015.
看護英和辞典（常葉恵子，他，編）医学書院，1992.
医学大辞典 第 2 版（伊藤 正男，井村裕夫，高久史麿，編集），医学書院，2009.
ステッドマン医学大辞典改訂第 6 版（ステッドマン医学大辞典編集委員会，編），メジカルビュー社，2008
新英和大辞典第 6 版（竹林滋，他，編），研究社，2002 など
200 万語専門用語 英和・和英大辞典（春遍雀來，編），日中韓辞典研究所，2011

● 編著者

園城寺康子（おんじょうじ・やすこ）

津田塾大学大学院文学研究科修士課程修了
元 聖隷加看護大学教授
著書「看護英語読解 15 のポイント」（共著）（メジカルビュー社）
訳書「看護論文を英語で書く」（共訳）（医学書院）

川越栄子（かわごえ・えいこ）

神戸女学院大学大学院文学研究科修士課程修了
神戸女学院大学教授
大阪大学・神戸大学医学部非常勤講師
著書「看護英語読解 15 のポイント」（共著）（メジカルビュー社）
「耳から学ぶ楽しいナース英語」（共著）（講談社）
「Travelers' First Aid Kit」（単著）（センゲージラーニング株式会社）
「ニュースで読む医療英語」(編集，共著)（講談社）

● 英文校閲

Christine D. Kuramoto（倉本クリスティーン）

Pacific Lutheran University, BA（Ed）
University of Birmingham UK, MA TEFL/TESL
Hamamatsu University School of Medicine, Associate Professor

改訂新版
これだけは知っておきたい **看護英語の基本用語と表現**
Nursing Terms And Expressions Everybody Uses

2007年 3月 30日第1版第1刷発行
2016年 1月 10日改訂新版第1刷発行
2022年 3月 1日　　　　　　　第3刷発行

- **編　著**　　園城寺　康子　おんじょうじやすこ
　　　　　　　川越　栄子　かわごええいこ
- **英文校閲**　Christine D. Kuramoto
- **発行者**　　吉田富生
- **発行所**　　株式会社メジカルビュー社
　　　　　　　〒162-0845　東京都新宿区市谷本村町2-30
　　　　　　　電話　03(5228)2050（代表）
　　　　　　　ホームページ　http://www.medicalview.co.jp

　　　　　　　営業部　FAX 03(5228)2059
　　　　　　　　　　　E-mail　eigyo@medicalview.co.jp

　　　　　　　編集部　FAX 03(5228)2062
　　　　　　　　　　　E-mail　ed@medicalview.co.jp

- **印刷所**　　シナノ印刷株式会社

ISBN978-4-7583-0446-7　C3047

©MEDICAL VIEW, 2007 & 2016.　Printed in Japan

- 本書に掲載された著作物の複写・複製・転載・翻訳・データベースへの取り込みおよび送信（送信可能化権を含む）・上映・譲渡に関する許諾権は，(株)メジカルビュー社が保有しています。
- JCOPY 〈(社)出版者著作権管理機構　委託出版物〉
本書の無断複写は著作権法上での例外を除き禁じられています。複写される場合は，そのつど事前に，(社)出版者著作権管理機構（電話 03-5244-5088, FAX 03-5244-5089, e-mail：info@jcopy.or.jp）の許諾を得てください。
- 本書をコピー，スキャン，デジタルデータ化するなどの複製を無許諾で行う行為は，著作権法上での限られた例外（「私的使用のための複製」など）を除き禁じられています。大学，病院，企業などにおいて，研究活動，診療を含む業務上使用する目的で上記の行為を行うことは私的使用には該当せず違法です。また私的使用のためであっても，代行業者等の第三者に依頼して上記の行為を行うことは違法となります。